P9-DGE-916

EXERCISING FOR FITNESS

TIME LIFE BOOKS

Other Publications:

CLASSICS OF THE OLD WEST
THE EPIC OF FLIGHT
THE GOOD COOK
THE SEAFARERS
THE ENCYCLOPEDIA OF COLLECTIBLES
THE GREAT CITIES
WORLD WAR II
HOME REPAIR AND IMPROVEMENT
THE WORLD'S WILD PLACES
THE TIME-LIFE LIBRARY OF BOATING
HUMAN BEHAVIOR
THE ART OF SEWING
THE OLD WEST
THE EMERGENCE OF MAN
THE AMERICAN WILDERNESS
THE TIME-LIFE ENCYCLOPEDIA OF GARDENING
LIFE LIBRARY OF PHOTOGRAPHY
THIS FABULOUS CENTURY
FOODS OF THE WORLD
TIME-LIFE LIBRARY OF AMERICA
TIME-LIFE LIBRARY OF ART
GREAT AGES OF MAN
LIFE SCIENCE LIBRARY
THE LIFE HISTORY OF THE UNITED STATES
TIME READING PROGRAM
LIFE NATURE LIBRARY
LIFE WORLD LIBRARY

FAMILY LIBRARY:
HOW THINGS WORK IN YOUR HOME
THE TIME-LIFE BOOK OF THE FAMILY CAR
THE TIME-LIFE FAMILY LEGAL GUIDE
THE TIME-LIFE BOOK OF FAMILY FINANCE

EXERCISING FOR **FITNESS**

by C. P. Gilmore

AND THE EDITORS OF TIME-LIFE BOOKS

LIBRARY OF HEALTH / TIME-LIFE BOOKS / ALEXANDRIA, VIRGINIA

THE AUTHOR:
C. P. Gilmore, an exercise enthusiast and marathon runner, is the editor-in-chief of *Popular Science*. A writer and radio and television commentator on medicine and the sciences for more than 20 years, he is the winner of many awards, including the Albert Lasker Award for Medical Writing. He has served as a member of the New York Heart Association Committee on Exercise.

THE CONSULTANTS:
William D. McArdle is professor of physical education at Queens College in New York City and the co-author of three books on physical fitness: *Getting in Shape; Nutrition, Weight Control, and Exercise;* and *Exercise Physiology: Food, Energy and Human Performance.*

Dr. Allan J. Ryan has been professor of rehabilitation medicine at the University of Wisconsin and editor-in-chief of *The Physician and Sportsmedicine,* a journal devoted to the treatment of injuries in sport. He is also the author of two books on the subject and has been a consultant to the President's Council on Physical Fitness and Sports.

For information about any Time-Life book, please write:
Reader Information, Time-Life Books,
541 North Fairbanks Court, Chicago, Illinois 60611.

©1981 Time-Life Books Inc. All rights reserved.
No part of this book may be reproduced in any form or by any electronic or mechanical means, including information storage and retrieval devices or systems, without prior written permission from the publisher except that brief passages may be quoted for reviews.

Second printing.
Published simultaneously in Canada.
School and library distribution by Silver Burdett Company, Morristown, New Jersey.

TIME-LIFE is a trademark of Time Incorporated U.S.A.

Library of Congress Cataloguing in Publication Data
Gilmore, Clarence Percy, 1926-
    Exercising for fitness.
    (Library of Health)
    Bibliography: p.
    Includes index.
    1. Exercise. 2. Physical fitness.
    I. Time-Life Books. II. Title. III. Series.
GV481.G5   613.7'1   80-25815
ISBN 0-8094-3756-2
ISBN 0-8094-3755-4 (lib. bdg.)
ISBN 0-8094-3754-6 (rctail cd.)

Time-Life Books Inc. is a wholly owned subsidiary of
TIME INCORPORATED

FOUNDER: Henry R. Luce 1898-1967

Editor-in-Chief: Henry Anatole Grunwald
President: J. Richard Munro
Chairman of the Board: Ralph P. Davidson
Executive Vice President: Clifford J. Grum
Chairman, Executive Committee: James R. Shepley
Editorial Director: Ralph Graves
Group Vice President, Books: Joan D. Manley
Vice Chairman: Arthur Temple

TIME-LIFE BOOKS INC.

MANAGING EDITOR: Jerry Korn
Executive Editor: David Maness
Assistant Managing Editors: Dale M. Brown (planning), George Constable, Martin Mann, John Paul Porter, Gerry Schremp (acting)
Art Director: Tom Suzuki
Chief of Research: David L. Harrison
Director of Photography: Robert G. Mason
Assistant Art Director: Arnold C. Holeywell
Assistant Chief of Research: Carolyn L. Sackett
Assistant Director of Photography: Dolores A. Littles

CHAIRMAN: John D. McSweeney
President: Carl G. Jaeger
Executive Vice Presidents: John Steven Maxwell, David J. Walsh
Vice Presidents: George Artandi (comptroller); Stephen L. Bair (legal counsel); Peter G. Barnes; Nicholas Benton (public relations); John L. Canova; Beatrice T. Dobie (personnel); Carol Flaumenhaft (consumer affairs); James L. Mercer (Europe/South Pacific); Herbert Sorkin (production); Paul R. Stewart (marketing)

LIBRARY OF HEALTH

Editorial Staff for *Exercising for Fitness*
Editor: William Frankel
Assistant Editor: Lee Hassig
Designer: Albert Sherman
Chief Researcher: Phyllis K. Wise
Picture Editor: Peggy L. Sawyer
Text Editors: Paul N. Mathless, David Thiemann
Staff Writers: Peter Kaufman, C. Tyler Mathisen
Researchers: Trudy W. Pearson and Maria Zacharias (principals), Judy D. French, Judith W. Shanks
Assistant Designer: Cynthia T. Richardson
Editorial Assistant: Shirley Fong Ash
Special Contributors: Peggy Eastman and Barbara Hicks

EDITORIAL PRODUCTION
Production Editor: Feliciano Madrid
Operations Manager: Gennaro C. Esposito, Gordon E. Buck (assistant)
Quality Control: Robert L. Young (director), James J. Cox (assistant), Daniel J. McSweeney, Michael G. Wight (associates)
Art Coordinator: Anne B. Landry
Copy Staff: Susan B. Galloway (chief), Margery duMond, Stephen G. Hyslop, Celia Beattie
Picture Department: Rebecca C. Christoffersen
Traffic: Kimberly K. Lewis

Correspondents: Elisabeth Kraemer (Bonn); Margot Hapgood, Dorothy Bacon, Lesley Coleman (London); Susan Jonas, Lucy T. Voulgaris (New York); Maria Vincenza Aloisi, Josephine du Brusle (Paris); Ann Natanson (Rome).
Valuable assistance was also provided by: Mirka Gondicas (Athens); Ken Huff (Detroit); Judy Aspinall (London); Marcia Gauger (New Delhi); Carolyn T. Chubet, Miriam Hsia, Christina Lieberman (New York); Marcel Brandao (Rio de Janeiro); Mimi Murphy (Rome).

CONTENTS

CHAPTER 1

Active life—healthy life

Help for the heart
Cutting down on dead weight
A psychological lift
Who should exercise
Sustaining the effort

All across West Germany, mounted at street corners and nailed to tree trunks along wooded trails, bright green-and-yellow signs mark the places where joggers assemble for their regularly scheduled runs.

In Paris, the 1961 running of the Cross du Figaro, a jogging race through the Bois de Boulogne, had 2,500 entrants; eight years later the number had ballooned to almost 36,000. The New York Marathon counted only 126 contestants for its first running in 1970; by 1979 there were more than 13,000.

In Finland, exercisers ski cross-country six or seven months of the year. Thousands of Finns log more than 300 miles on skis each year, traveling some of the distance on lighted courses built to lengthen the short days of the Northern winter. Urho Kekkonen, Finland's durable President, trekked about 600 miles on skis during his 79th year.

In the United States, some 34 million people engage in regular, active walking for exercise; 17 million run. In some places, the running boom overtaxed the available facilities. The indoor track at a Boston YMCA became so crowded at one point that an official claimed, ''You run in step or you get killed.'' The city manager of Los Altos Hills, California, complained that joggers ''take over the streets on weekends, sometimes 100 strong, five and six abreast, and refuse to get out of the traffic lanes.''

In America, as in other nations, the burgeoning popularity of exercise has many faces.

● Active participation in sports that demand physical fitness has expanded greatly. When Olga Korbut of the Soviet Union won the 1972 Olympic Gold Medal in gymnastics, there were an estimated 50,000 youngsters in the United States taking part in this sport. Less than a decade later, the figure had risen to close to a million.

● In 10 years bookstores doubled the shelves devoted to physical activity; they became jammed with volumes on everything from roller skating to jumping rope. The National Sporting Goods Association reported that annual sales of athletic equipment increased from $3.6 billion to more than $5 billion in two years.

● Membership in the YMCA increased 16 per cent in a recent decade; attendance at exercise classes conducted by the Y jumped 26 per cent in five years. In 1980 more than 4,000 health clubs specialized in physical fitness.

● Hundreds of companies across America, following the lead of Japanese industry, began to provide the time and place for employees to exercise. The American Association of Fitness Directors in Business and Industry—an organization made up of the people who run these employee programs—had more than 300 members only four years after its founding in 1974.

● Hotels installed exercise facilities. The Chicago Marriott, for example, provided courts for paddle tennis, an indoor pool, weight-lifting apparatus, a treadmill for running, and other facilities. The Sheraton chain set up jogging courses at seven of its hotels.

Clearly, something was going on. ''We believe,'' said Richard O. Keelor of the President's Council on Physical

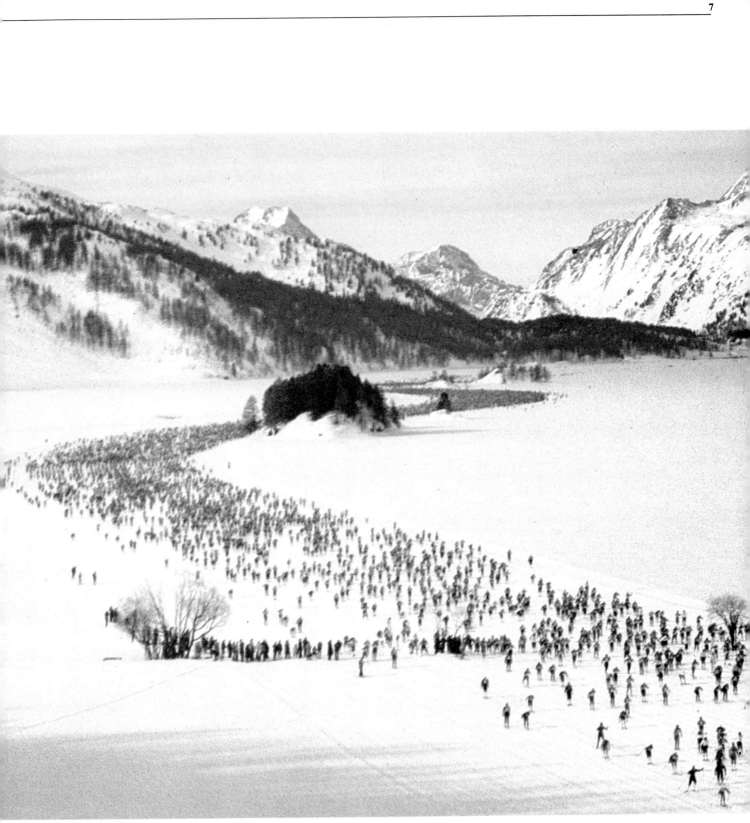

A river of skiers starts Switzerland's Engadin Skimarathon,
an event that draws growing crowds of people who exercise for
fitness. The annual competition enrolled 945 cross-country
skiers for its first running in 1969; for its 10th, when this picture
was taken, the 26-mile race attracted more than 12,000
entrants, 90 per cent of whom crossed the finish line.

Fitness and Sports, "that America is going through a physical fitness renaissance." The statistics bear out his contention. A sampling survey by the polling firm of Louis Harris and Associates in 1978 found that 59 per cent of Americans 18 years of age and older spent two and a half hours or more each week participating in some sort of regular exercise; in a similar survey taken two decades earlier, the figure was only 24 per cent.

While most people are content to exercise moderately for a flatter belly, a springier step and a more alert feeling, about 15 per cent of the regular exercisers were classified by the Harris survey as "high actives"—they spent more than five hours a week engaged in vigorous exercise. And some enthusiasts were achieving levels of fitness all but unknown except in competitive athletes.

For example, when 52-year-old John Huckaby of Lee Center, New York, learned that he had an ailing heart and high blood pressure, he began walking to improve his health, and then switched to running. After six years "the Incredible Huck," as he called himself, had worked up to about eight miles every day during his lunch break and six miles three nights a week with a YMCA group. During 1978 he logged about 3,000 miles, including 12 marathons of 26.2 miles each—he ran two of them on successive days—and the 50-mile John F. Kennedy Memorial race, held annually in Boonsboro, Maryland. During the same six years, Huckaby lost 85 pounds, cut his blood pressure in half and eliminated the irregularities in his heartbeat as well as the angina chest pain he had experienced.

Yet the same statistics that proved there was a fitness boom

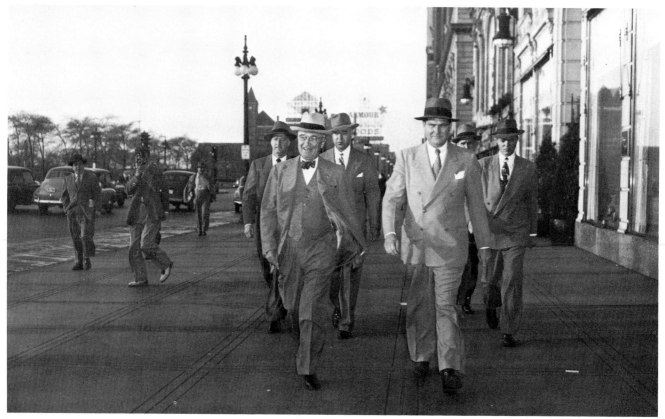

Journalists and Secret Service men tag after President Harry S. Truman—66 years old when this picture was taken—on a morning walk in Chicago. Truman covered one and a half miles each day, striding at a purposeful 120 paces a minute. "If you are going to walk for your physical benefit," he observed, "it is necessary that you walk as if you are going someplace."

also demonstrated that many people were almost exclusively sedentary. In the United States the Harris study that found all those exercising Americans also found the corollary: 41 per cent did no regular exercise, and many of them, apparently, never did anything more physically demanding than walking from the television to the refrigerator for another beer during a commercial.

In Israel as recently as the mid-1970s, only 35 per cent of the adult population participated in any kind of regular exercise. In Italy the percentage of people who exercise is even lower. England boasts only a few per cent more swimmers than dart players.

In Germany many people believe "that nature and fresh air make them fit," began a report by the German Sports Association on physical fitness there, but not if exposure to the outdoors requires much effort. Germans "pack a picnic basket in the car," the report continued, "drive to a parking place in a forest and sit on the grass 30 feet from the car. There they wolf down a giant helping of potato salad, empty a few bottles of beer and return home with the reassuring feeling that once again they have restored themselves to the bosom of nature."

Most people will not walk even a few steps if they can ride. Just three blocks from the New York Hospital is a subway stop that is used by many members of the hospital staff. On any morning at about 8:45 they crowd the street exit of the subway, waiting for a bus to carry them to the hospital. Often the wait is longer than the five minutes that it would take to walk. It is doubtful that the idea of walking ever occurred to most of them.

A striking example of this prejudice against exertion was provided when two of the four elevators in an apartment building broke down. A small, impatient crowd accumulated in the lobby, ignoring the stairs nearby and waiting for one of the two functioning cars to appear. One woman, who seemed especially annoyed by the inconvenience, muttered loudly about the appalling maintenance of the building. When after perhaps five minutes an elevator finally appeared, the crowd jammed in and the complaining woman pushed the button—for the second floor.

It is tempting to surmise that the difference between those who do not exercise and those who do lies in divergent opinions about the value of physical activity, that exercisers pursue benefits that their sedentary counterparts feel are not worth the effort. However, such an assumption is incorrect. Most people, whether they exercise regularly or not, believe that exercise is good for them, promoting the fitness that characterizes generally sound health. It does. But there is great confusion about what constitutes beneficial exercise, how much of it is necessary to be effective and what health benefits it can convey.

One popular book maintained that 10 easy minutes of calisthenics three times a week was plenty of exercise for anyone, and among the Americans surveyed by the Harris firm, about half felt that normal everyday activities give all the exercise anyone needs. For most people in the industrialized world, this is not true. Substantial numbers of people also believe that golf and tennis doubles provide enough exercise for fitness. Neither ordinarily does.

At the opposite extreme are exaggerated and misleading claims made by exercise evangelists. One doctor, himself a runner, asserted that no one who has ever completed a marathon has died of a heart attack; the fact is that many runners—including marathon runners—have been felled by heart attack.

The truth about exercise lies somewhere between these extreme opinions. No single type of exercise serves all purposes; rather there is a variety of activities—including some enjoyable sports—that enable any person to match his capacities and preferences to his needs. Exercise can strengthen muscles, including the vital heart muscle. It is almost essential in getting rid of excess fat in order to control weight and shape the body into pleasing contours. It gives physical stamina and pliability so that the everyday chores of living can be performed without tiring effort or injurious strain. Somehow, exercise provides relaxation and seems to promote mental well-being.

Exactly how these benefits are achieved by exercise—and to what degree—is still a subject of much debate. There is a great difference between what scientists know and what

The safety bicycle: a two-wheeled tonic

"For the sedentary," declared *Bicycling for Ladies,* a manual of the 1890s, "the bicycle seems to work wonders. The organs of digestion are stimulated, the appetite improves, and the mind responds readily." The healthful benefits thus foreseen helped set off a fad that sent millions of cyclists whizzing down streets and country roads in Europe and America, a craze rekindled 75 years later by renewed awareness of the value of exercise.

The 19th Century enthusiasm for cycling stemmed from an invention, the safety bicycle. Until it appeared, cycling was often a risky and unpleasant venture. Few cared to master the preceding type of bicycle, the penny-farthing, with a huge front wheel that raised the rider several feet off the ground and made the vehicle virtually unmanageable. The safety bicycle had smaller wheels of equal size that kept the rider's feet reassuringly within reach of the ground, and it came with pneumatic tires, which softened what had been a bone-shaking ride on solid wheels.

Because the new machine opened the sport to nearly everyone, it had more impact on social custom than on health. Young men too impoverished to keep a horse could court young women who lived across town. And the ladies shed their corsets for the freedom to breathe that strenuous pedaling demanded. Faster than ever before, children eluded parents' watchful eyes. Clergymen, alarmed by crowds of cyclists enjoying Sunday morning spins instead of listening to sermons, predicted the damnation of such defilers of the Sabbath.

Doctors, meanwhile, debated whether the activity aided or harmed health. Some pointed to cycling as the cause of ills ranging from insanity to muscle twitch. Another malady allegedly peculiar to the sport—and certainly new to science—was bicycle hump, a misshapen back said to be induced by the rump-high, shoulders-low posture of the more speed-intoxicated cyclists.

The 19th Century medical consensus was that such bike-related afflictions as existed were limited mostly to zealots. Cycling in moderation, most doctors felt, strengthened the lungs, toned the muscles and—in a strikingly prescient forecast of modern opinion—may even have helped the heart.

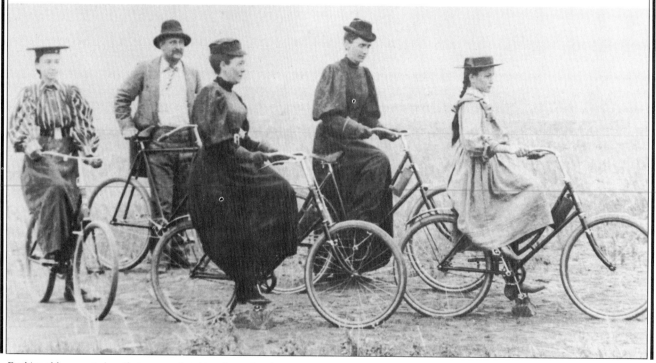

Fashionably mounted on their new safety bicycles, a South Dakota family tours the countryside in the 1890s, the years of the initial bicycle boom. It began in 1891, peaked in five years and faded by 1900, not to revive for more than seven decades.

they only suspect about how the human body responds to exercise and how an active life contributes to good physical and mental health.

Help for the heart

That regular exercise confers healthful benefits seems to be documented. Professor A. H. Ismail of Purdue University studied the medical records of 44 men for four years and found that medical expenses for the sedentary members of the group averaged $400 a year, but doctors' bills for regular exercisers added up to only half that amount.

A study conducted in Sweden between 1958 and 1967 produced similar results. During that 10-year period, a group of 88 exercisers were ill for a total of 4,673 days, an average of about five days per person per year. In contrast, an equal number of nonactive people, comparable to the first group in age and sex, counted up 13,478 sick days, nearly three times as many as the exercisers.

Scientists must be careful how they interpret such research. The studies that show a lower frequency of illness among exercisers than nonexercisers seem to demonstrate that exercise makes people healthier, but they might prove only that people who exercise regularly do so because they are healthier to begin with.

One example of the difficulty of proving that exercise results in better health is the tenuous connection between exercise and reduced risk of heart disease. Physiologists have demonstrated to everyone's satisfaction that a certain type of regular exercise (Chapters 2 and 3) brings about a number of changes in the heart and circulatory system. The heart, for example, acquires the capacity to pump more blood with each beat than it did before. Blood pressure generally drops slightly; the resting pulse rate slows—indeed, the heart may beat as many as 13 million fewer times per year. As Dr. Gabe Mirkin, who specializes in the medical effects of exercise, said, ''The heart becomes like a low-mileage used car; it takes longer to wear out.'' Laboratory tests on rats bear him out. Rodents that have been exercised live 25 per cent longer than their unexercised cousins.

But none of this evidence, intriguing as it may be, addresses directly the question of whether exercise protects against heart disease or extends the lives of humans. Most people—and a lot of them are experts in the field—believe that it does. Yet the surprising fact is that while thousands of researchers have devoted immense sums of money and countless hours over several decades to this question, it has not been answered conclusively.

An impressive amount of circumstantial evidence has piled up, but it is subject to criticism on one point or another.

Dr. Ralph Paffenbarger of Stanford University kept statistics on groups of exercisers and compared these figures with those for similar groups of nonexercisers to see if there are differences between groups in the incidence of heart attacks. After keeping track of 6,300 longshoremen for 22 years, he found that among those with the more active jobs the incidence of heart attack was half of what it was for longshoremen employed in more sedentary positions, even when other factors affecting the heart were taken into account. In another study Dr. Paffenbarger examined the health records of 16,936 Harvard alumni from the classes of 1916 to 1950 and divided the subjects into two groups: those who exercised enough to burn up 2,000 calories a week (the number expended in about three hours of running) and those who consumed fewer than 2,000 calories a week in exercise. Those in the high-exercise group had 36 per cent fewer heart attacks than those in the other group. Much other research over the years yielded similar patterns.

More thought-provoking is a study in five American cities of 651 male survivors of heart attacks. They were randomly divided into two more or less equal groups. The subjects in one group agreed to participate in a regimen of exercise as part of their rehabilitation; those in the other group agreed not to exercise regularly. The researchers found that after three years men in the sedentary control group died of heart attacks at a rate eight times as high as that of the men in the exercising group.

It is hard to avoid the conclusion that exercise can decrease the probability of heart attack. But neither this five-city study nor the Paffenbarger research conclusively establishes anything of the kind. The heart attack victims were sick men, and what exercise accomplished for them cannot logically be extrapolated to determine what it might do for healthy people. Dr. Paffenbarger's work and the comparisons of medical costs among exercisers and sedentary individuals suffer from the same weakness—strenuous physical activity may only reflect good health, not create it.

Indeed, there is evidence to support this point of view. Researchers at Peter Bent Brigham Hospital in Boston and Harvard Medical School examined the family histories of a large group of marathon runners and found that the incidence of coronary heart disease among their fathers was 40 per cent of that among the fathers of nonrunners. So it is possible that those who chose to achieve the high levels of fitness necessary for marathon running had healthier genes to begin with, passed on to them by their fathers.

Less equivocal evidence that exercise might forestall heart attack comes from research into the effects on the heart of cholesterol, a fat used by the body as a vital part of cell walls and as raw material for sex hormones and bile acids. It has been known for years that a high level of cholesterol in the blood is associated with an increased risk of heart attack. Cholesterol does not travel alone in the blood but must first be combined with proteins to form other substances called lipoproteins. Lipoproteins come in several varieties, but most of the cholesterol occurs in two of them: high-density lipoproteins (HDLs) and low-density lipoproteins (LDLs).

In 1975, while trying to establish whether the level of cholesterol in the blood could be used to predict the amount of cholesterol in the rest of the body, the British physician-brothers Norman and George Miller posed a hypothesis that was to have important consequences. On the basis of their compilation of about 100 observations published by other researchers, the Millers reported that in people whose levels of HDL were high in comparison with their levels of LDL, the total amount of cholesterol was depressed. It seemed, they suggested, as if HDLs were rich in cholesterol not because they were carrying this dangerous substance to deposit it around the body, but because they were acting like garbage trucks to help the body get rid of it.

The researchers theorized that high levels of HDL might be associated with a reduced risk of heart attack. They pointed out that women, whose blood contains more HDLs than that of men, have a lower risk of heart attack. Furthermore, certain ethnic groups with high heart attack rates, such as the Scots, seem to have small quantities of HDL; certain groups suffering few heart attacks, such as Jamaican farmers and Greenland Eskimos, tend to have greater amounts of HDL. Such evidence has led most experts to accept the idea that the amount of this lipoprotein in a person's blood is more important than the total amount of cholesterol in indicating the likelihood that he will have a heart attack.

At about the same time as the Millers' discovery in Britain, Peter Wood, a biochemist at Stanford University, uncovered another important clue. Wood, who had been a distance runner for years, often used his own blood in his research on heart disease. He had noticed that its content of HDL was much higher than that in most samples he dealt with. He decided to see if the same was true of other people who exercised as much as he did.

Wood and his colleagues selected a group of 45 male runners between 35 and 59 years of age and compared their blood with that of 45 relatively sedentary men in the same age range. They found that the sedentary subjects averaged about .45 milligram of HDL per milliliter (.0075 ounce per pint) of blood. But for the runners the average was .65 milligram per milliliter.

Wood's experiment demonstrated only that runners possessed high HDL levels, not that running had produced them. But subsequent experiments by researchers at Duke University in Durham, North Carolina, indicated that sedentary men and women can increase the amount of HDL in their blood by an average of .17 milligram per milliliter of blood—about the same quantity as the difference in HDL levels between runners and nonrunners in Wood's observations—after 10 weeks of running or similar exercise such as bicycling or swimming.

Research completed in 1979 by a team of investigators at the Methodist Hospital in Houston, Texas, carries the work of Wood and the Duke University team one step further. This study looked at three groups: inactive individuals, joggers

Fanciful claims for reducing gimmicks

Exercising to lose weight and firm the body demands hard work, will power and time. Many would-be reducers try to find an easier way—and buy garments and gadgets that government agencies have held to be useless or even hazardous.

Among the most common of these gimmicks are garments such as the ones in the advertisements reproduced at right. Made of material that traps heat and seals in moisture, they are supposed to provide permanent weight loss. Medical authorities say they do not. By preventing the evaporation of sweat, they cause increased sweating—which rids the body not of fat, but of fluid; the fluids lost are soon replenished by a few glasses of water. To make matters worse, some of the products can aggravate high blood pressure and heart trouble by squeezing tissues so that blood circulation is restricted.

The reducing suits pictured here have been banned from the mails, and sale of the electrical device on the following pages was restricted to physicians by court order. These legal actions do not prevent other devices like them from being sold in the future. There is only one certain protection against exaggerated claims for any reducing aid: Remember that there is no easy way to lose weight.

Extravagant claims fill an array of advertisements for apparel that is supposed to cause weight loss without exercise or diet. All four products have been banned from the United States mails.

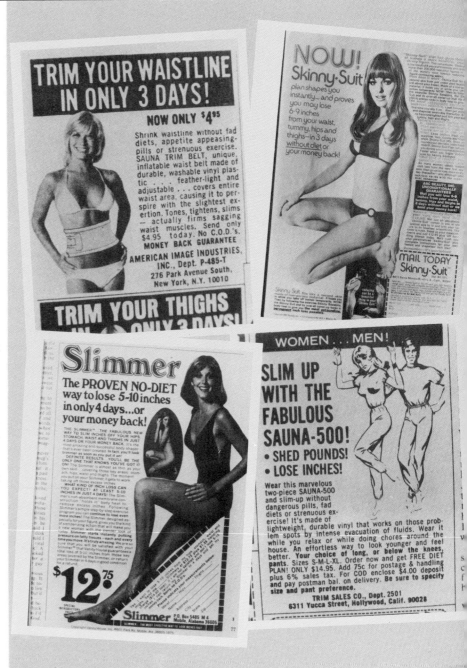

Danger from an electric machine

A grim chapter in the history of so-called effortless exercise devices was written by the RelaxAcizor, an electric muscle stimulator whose plug was pulled in 1970 by a federal judge. The device consisted of a control box, a belt to be strapped around the waist, hips or shoulders, and pads to be placed wherever weight loss was desired. It delivered electrical shocks to the muscles, forcing them to contract 40 times a minute.

Said one infuriated customer: "I spent $249.50 on this thing, and I was supposed to lose half a pound an hour. I put it on every day for ninety days. I didn't lose anything—except $249.50."

Other users had more sinister complaints. They reported muscle pain, skin disorders and spells of anxiety. The Food and Drug Administration found that the dangers of the RelaxAcizor were, if anything, even worse than the reports, and eventually won a court injunction against its sale to the general public. After hearing expert medical testimony, Judge William P. Gray listed 30 maladies the machine could cause, including back pain, breathing difficulty and miscarriage. "Use of the RelaxAcizor," he concluded, "may jeopardize the health and even the life of the user in ways that may not be apparent to him."

Claims of effortless exercise for men and thinner hips for women (right) helped sell an electrical muscle stimulator called the RelaxAcizor to 400,000 buyers at prices up to $450. After government action prohibited the sale of the dangerous machine except to physicians, warnings (far right) were displayed in post offices.

EFFORTLESS EXERCISE FOR THE MODERN MAN

Modern man is busy. Yet — he often needs exercise — and most usually exercise of a specific body area, like the waist-abdomen region. Many men, nowadays, are "chained" to a desk or an office for a good portion of their day. It is increasingly difficult for these men to take the time for the exercise schedule necessary to maintain their muscle tone. And, the waistline and abdomen are usually the areas that show this lack of exercise. Yet modern man, along with his rather sedentary existence, is expected to look "in shape".

How does the busy modern man reduce the size of his expanding waistline and abdomen? The answer for many men is a remarkable device called Relax-A-cizor. Relax-A-cizor exercises and tightens the muscles of this area while you rest or read. There's no physical effort . . . and its use takes a mere ½ hour a day!

Many men lack good muscle tone because they don't get enough exercise. Relax-A-cizor gives effortless, concentrated exercise to such body areas as the waistline and abdomen. Regular use causes this area to reduce in size measurably to the extent these muscles lack tone because of insufficient exercise. And the less the muscle tone, the greater the degree of size reduction.

Reduce Size of HIPS!

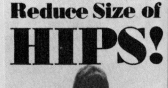

How are YOUR hips? A bit too "hippy"? Waistline and tummy sort of "stretched out of shape," too? Take heart. NOW — there's a way. A wonderful no-work way.

Relax-A-cizor "effortless exercise" reduces the SIZE of hips, waistline, tummy and thighs while you REST at home.

NO WEIGHT LOSS. Relax-A-cizor is different. Completely different. Luxurious muscle toning . . . without a whit of effort!

Here's how it works: Many women lack good muscle tone because they don't get enough exercise. Relax-A-cizor gives effortless, concentrated exercise to such figure areas as hips, waistline, abdomen and thighs. Regular use causes these areas to reduce in size measurably to the extent these muscles lack tone because of insufficient exercise. And the less the muscle tone the greater the degree of size reduction.

FREE! Find out what Relax-A-cizor can do for YOU! Send for your free copy of "Your Figure" by Burton Skiles. No cost. No obligation.   © Relax-A-cizor 1967

RelaxAcizor.

PRINCIPAL OFFICES: NEW YORK, N. Y., 575 Madison Ave., MU 8-4690/CHICAGO, ILL., 29 E. Madison St., ST 2-5680/LOS ANGELES, CALIFORNIA, 980 No. La Cienega Blvd., OL 5-8000/

PUBLIC BEWARE!

WARNING AGAINST RELAXACIZORS

All persons who use a Relaxacizor device for muscle exercise and other purposes are hereby advised and warned that the device has been found to be dangerous to health by a United States District Court. Relaxacizor devices have been distributed since 1949, and approximately 400,000 units have been sold.

The Court found that the Relaxacizor may:

1. Aggravate many medical conditions in susceptible persons;

2. Have a serious potential for damage to the heart and other vital body organs; and

3. Be capable of causing a miscarriage, and otherwise may jeopardize the health and even the life of the user.

For further information write to:
U.S. Department of Health,
Education, and Welfare
Public Health Service
Food and Drug Administration
5600 Fishers Lane
Rockville, Maryland 20852

who reported covering an average of 11 miles per week, and runners who averaged 40 miles per week and had completed one marathon within the preceding 12 months. The joggers and marathon runners alike had higher levels of HDL in their blood than the sedentary group, and the marathon runners had more HDL than the joggers. To the investigators this result suggested that HDL levels increase in proportion to the distance run.

On another front, the researchers at Duke University found that regular, vigorous exercise alters the chemical composition of the blood in such a way that it is better able to dissolve blood clots. Because clots in an artery are believed to trigger some heart attacks, strokes and other circulatory diseases by cutting off circulation to the heart, brain or some other vital organ, the change in the blood induced by exercise

may also give some protection against such disorders.

It is studies such as these that have convinced an ever-increasing number of scientists that exercise is valuable in promoting good health, even though conclusive proof is yet to come. Dr. Paffenbarger, one of the strongest proponents of this view, flatly stated his belief that the association between exercise and lowered risk of heart attack "cannot be attributed merely to an inclination toward exercise among those who are naturally fit. I'm convinced," he said, "that activity per se lowers the risk of heart attack, and the more vigorous the level of exercise, the better the protection." If this is the case, then physical activity will on an average prolong life, for heart attack is among the principal causes of death in the industrialized world.

Although there is yet no direct proof that exercise is connected to the resistance of the human heart and circulatory system to disease, other links between health and exercise are more firmly established. Such a relationship is the one between physical activity and obesity.

Cutting down on dead weight

No one doubts that excess fat impairs health; life insurance companies, drawing on comparisons of weight and mortality over more than a century, have made most people aware of the dangers of overweight. One exhaustive study of 5,127 Americans showed that if you weigh 20 per cent more than the ideal weight for your height and sex, your chances of succumbing to a heart attack are tripled.

In most of the industrialized world, men and women have become heavier in recent times. In the United States, for example, the average woman between the ages of 35 and 44 was six pounds heavier in 1980 than her counterpart 20 years earlier. Men of the same age were eight pounds heavier. Yet many Americans decreased their food consumption within a similar period—from 2,250 calories a day in 1965 to 1,970 calories in 1977—and there is no sign that the trend has reversed.

That people become fatter even as they eat less has a simple explanation: Physical activity, which consumes most of the calories in food, has declined faster than calorie con-

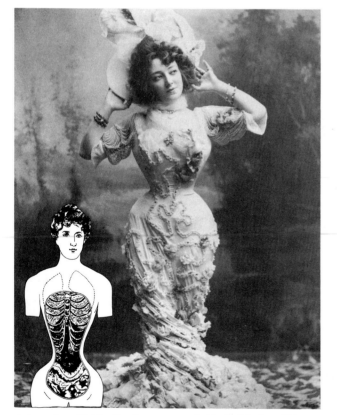

Actress Anna Held epitomizes a womanly ideal of the late 19th Century: a plump body given shape by a viselike corset. Attacking this unhealthful way of achieving fashionable proportions, reformers used pictures (inset) of women's bodies grotesquely compressed by the garments. This artist erred in detail if not in message—corsets squeeze organs upward, not downward.

sumption. When the intake of calories is greater than the expenditure in activity, the surplus becomes fat. Most Americans and Europeans now earn a living behind a desk, ride everywhere they go and watch television during most of their leisure hours. Housewives tend to be a bit more active than their husbands but not enough to make much difference, for they no longer wash clothes by hand, beat carpets or perform other heavy work.

If a sedentary life puts on pounds, then it stands to reason that exercise ought to help take them off. Yet for years the myth was perpetuated that exercise is of little help in weight control. Conventional wisdom held that not only does it take huge amounts of exercise to work off any significant amount of fat, but that exercise is to some degree self-defeating because it makes you hungry so you will eat more, restoring the excess that you worked so hard to shed.

There is some truth to both contentions, but they must be seen in context. Although considerable exercise is required to decrease weight noticeably, there is no rule that it must all be done at once. Physiologists determined, for example, that a 150-pound person walking at a rate of 2.5 miles an hour—a leisurely pace—for one hour each day will in a year burn enough calories to shed 22 pounds of fat. The amount of exercise that Dr. Paffenbarger found to give such dramatic protection from heart attack—2,000 calories' worth a week—could take off almost 30 pounds in a year. Thus even moderate exercise on a regular basis can be very effective in reducing weight.

The belief that exercisers counterbalance any weight worked off by eating more arises from an undeniable fact: Vigorous exercisers do eat more. (During America's bicentennial celebration in 1976, signs appeared in restaurants offering travelers their fill of food for a low price; in establishments along a transcontinental bicycle route marked for the bicentennial, many of the signs read: ''All you can eat—$3.95. Bikers—$4.95.'') On the other hand, moderate exercise may suppress appetite in those who are sedentary and overweight, helping to equalize food intake and energy output for overeaters.

But regardless of whether a person is one in whom exercise

increases appetite or decreases it, weight usually declines with regular exertion. Many studies have demonstrated that active people weigh far less than their lethargic counterparts. Men who exercise are 20 per cent less heavy than men who do not. Women who exercise regularly are 30 per cent lighter than women who rarely exert themselves. Furthermore, most of the weight lost through exercise is in the form of fat; reducing by dieting alone also sacrifices lean muscle tissues that the body needs. One reason that women lose a larger percentage of their weight than men when they exercise is that more of a woman's weight is contributed by fat tissue; they have more to lose.

Reducing with exercise almost always gives women and men better-looking figures. The reason is simple. Exercise decreases weight by eliminating fat, and most fat accumu-

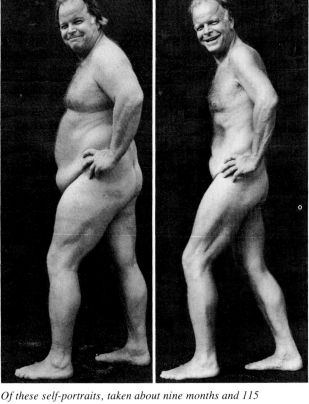

Of these self-portraits, taken about nine months and 115 pounds apart, New York photographer Bob Adelman wrote: ''I look like I just hatched out of that 305-pound blob.'' To shed the excess weight, Adelman combined psychological ploys to control overeating with a regimen of increasingly vigorous exercise that eventually had him running several miles a day.

lates around the middle of the body, at the waist and hips (and in women, in the thighs and arms). Thus the weight taken off by exercise does not cause the body to shrink in overall size; instead, it changes the body's shape, toward the slim form that society favors.

In addition to eliminating fat, exercise contributes to the slim form in another way—by strengthening muscles. Stronger stomach and back muscles lift a sagging middle and improve posture, both of which enhance appearance. They also provide the strength everyone needs to cope with day-to-day activities—to wrestle a suitcase through a vacation trip, to lug an easy chair into a new position, to carry a large potted plant from the porch to the house.

If the physiological benefits claimed for exercise are real, as seems likely, and not simply another way of saying that healthy people enjoy physical activity while sickly ones do not, then exercise is as important as a nutritious diet to the longevity of mankind. It may also be important to mental well-being. The awareness of such a connection between the body and the mind is relatively new.

Since antiquity, exercise and sports have been extolled as the means toward a sound body to shelter and nurture a sound mind. Among the Greeks and Romans and in later civilizations, mental soundness was the reward for intellectual labor just as corporeal soundness was the product of physical exertion.

At the turn of the 19th Century, however, the rigid barrier between mental and physical began to break down under the probings of psychologists and psychiatrists. On the one hand, they demonstrated that an individual's mental condition, if he is depressed or otherwise disturbed, can precipitate disease or worsen one already in progress. On the other, more recently they have begun to collect evidence that physical activity, apart from its physiological implications, may also produce salutary effects on a person's state of mind.

A psychological lift

Practically anyone who exercises regularly has good things to say about the ways that it has improved his feelings. Not everyone reports the same effects, but as a group exercisers assert that they have a more positive outlook on life, concentrate better and cope with problems more effectively. They say that they feel more assertive, think more creatively and are more self-confident.

More dramatic mental benefits have also been observed, for exercise seems to help the psychologically disturbed. A leading advocate of exercise as a treatment for emotional disorders is Dr. Thaddeus Kostrubala, a psychiatrist who founded the International Association of Running Therapies in San Diego. Dr. Kostrubala developed an interest in the psychologically therapeutic value of exercise in a roundabout way. When, at the age of 46, he became concerned about his own increasing obesity, he decided to participate in a hospital exercise program designed for patients recuperating from heart attacks. "As we progressed I began to notice not only physical but psychological changes in the patients," he said. "Well, like most psychiatrists, I had some patients of my own with whom I was just up against the wall—we were making absolutely no progress in treatment. So I decided to try running with them."

Dr. Kostrubala put his patients on a schedule of running three times a week, followed by group psychotherapy. Changes, he said, "were remarkable." Those with depression had fewer symptoms. A schizophrenic man could be taken off the medication he had needed, and a young woman with anorexia nervosa—a serious condition in which patients refuse food and can literally starve themselves to death—resumed eating. "Also," he continued, "destructive relationships were alleviated or ended."

Dr. Kostrubala admitted, however, that his observations may suffer from hidden biases and that not all his patients have responded to what he called running therapy. But he was satisfied that this treatment worked for many people and he included it among the choices of therapy that he continues to offer his patients.

The apparent effectiveness of exercise in relieving symptoms of mental disorders has prompted laboratory studies of the phenomenon. In one experiment at the University of Virginia, more than 500 students were asked to take tests formulated to draw a more reliable picture of a person's

A Fairfax County fire fighter, burdened with more than 60 pounds of gear, runs from his truck during a proficiency drill. By the time he reaches the fire, his pulse may have soared to more than 180 beats a minute, better than twice its normal rate.

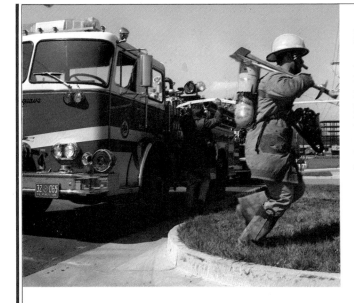

Fighting fire with fitness

Almost half the professional fire fighters killed in the line of duty in the 1970s in the United States died not from flame or smoke but from heart attacks. One reason became clear from tests of the physical condition of fire fighters in Los Angeles, Washington, D.C., and other cities: They were no more fit than the average sedentary American male, although their duties impose extreme demands. A fire fighter may have to race up stairs, with 60 pounds of gear and 70 pounds of hose and nozzle.

Among departments that began to require exercises was the Fairfax County, Virginia, Fire and Rescue Services, which in 1979 ordered each member to work with weights and run or cycle. Lieutenant Ken Jones, the medical-physical coordinator, observed "a department-wide decrease in weight and an increased lung capacity." Before the program, 24 of a sample of more than 100 of the Services' members failed a breathing test and 20 were overweight; after a year, five failed and nine were overweight.

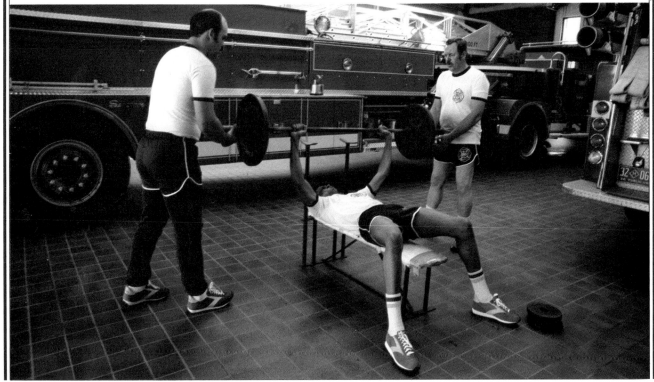

In the firehouse, one fire fighter lifts a barbell as two others stand by to support the 135-pound load if he tires. For aerobic exercise, the station's entire crew, less the radio operator, take the hook and ladder and the pumper to a nearby athletic field, where the fire fighters jog, ready to respond to a call.

feelings than can be obtained simply by asking him how he feels. The tests revealed that about 18 per cent of the students were depressed; the rest were normal. Some subjects in each group were then asked to jog regularly for 10 weeks; others were asked not to.

At the end of the experiment, psychological tests were administered again. The outlooks of depressed students who had done no exercise remained virtually the same, but among those who ran, symptoms of depression were substantially lowered. Students who ran five times a week showed more improvement than ones who exercised only three times a week. Participants whose depression scores had been normal before the experiment obtained even better scores after running. Another phase of the study indicated similar benefits among joggers, tennis players and wrestling-team members, but not among players of softball, a relatively slow-paced game.

Scientists do not know why exercise seems to have a beneficial effect on depression. It may be related to the fact that someone who is depressed generally feels better after successfully performing even one simple task, such as exercising for 10 weeks.

There may also be a chemical connection between exercise and alleviation of depression. Many researchers have found evidence that exercise promotes production in the brain of the hormone norepinephrine, which seems related to emotional stability. One such study, conducted in 1979 by Drs. Joel Dimsdale and Jonathan Moss at Massachusetts General Hospital in Boston, involved nine volunteers, all young physicians on the hospital staff. Each wore a portable blood-sampling device so that specimens of his blood could be taken during various activities. Exercise lasted four minutes and consisted of climbing and descending some 10 flights of stairs. By analyzing blood samples taken during exercise, the researchers discovered that the level of norepinephrine in the blood increased on the average by more than three times during the short bout of stair climbing.

Though this experiment ignored any short-term emotional effects that the higher levels of norepinephrine may have had on the volunteers, other studies indicate that people with balanced emotions seem to enjoy high levels of this hormone and of a similar one called epinephrine; depressed individuals have low levels. However, more research is needed to ascertain whether the hormone causes the mood change or the mood change alters the hormone level. Other theories contend that exercise affects mood by increasing blood flow to the brain, perhaps because the brain thrives on the extra oxygen and nutrients it receives.

Who should exercise

The psychological and physiological profits of exercise accrue to everyone, male and female, young and old. This fact has long been accepted, but it has not been acted upon. Until recently, regular, vigorous exercise—undertaken for its aid in promoting fitness—has been largely the province of men, and mainly men in their young to middle years. Only now is the importance of deliberate programs of activity for children, women and the elderly being recognized.

Children were thought to get enough exercise from play. That many of them do not is indicated by the alarming incidence of obesity in the young, caused generally by inactivity—most fat children eat less than slim ones but are much less active.

Women, too, have not engaged in exercise programs, but for different reasons. For one thing, women were wrongly discouraged by the idea of competing with men. In general men are taller, heavier and more extensively muscled—about 45 per cent of body weight is muscle in young men, as opposed to about 27 per cent in young women. Men have heavier and larger bones and less body fat. These differences put women at a disadvantage in most competitive sports. But when it comes to endurance, they come close. Women hold long-distance swimming records, and excel in races of 50 miles and longer.

Another belief that kept some women from vigorous exercise was the idea that it developed bulging, unfeminine muscles. This notion seems mistaken. Women's muscles can increase dramatically in strength while changing size hardly at all. Jack Wilmore, Professor of Physical Education at the University of Arizona, said that women increase muscle

*Attempting to gauge oxygen consumption, a researcher
takes the pulse of a Tarahumare pedaling a stationary
bicycle. Results were disappointing—the Indians would
not pedal fast enough for valid measurements.*

Indian runners of the Sierra Madre

For centuries running has been a way of life among the Tarahumare Indians of Mexico's Sierra Madre, a region too rug-
ged for burros but not for the vigorous Tarahumare. Most of
them go about their business at a jog instead of a walk, and
prodigious feats of endurance are a tradition. Around 1900,
one runner carried a message nearly 250 miles and returned
to his village in five days. It was once common for the Tarahumare to hunt deer by pursuing them day and night until the
animals collapsed in exhaustion. Today the tribe perpetuates
a custom of kickball races that may cover 100 miles or more
(below) and continue without pause for three days and nights.

Though tests to measure the Tarahumare's stamina *(right)*
have had only limited success—the Indians refuse to exhaust
themselves for medical research—physical examinations
have revealed low pulse rates and blood pressure, little fat,
and low cholesterol levels in the Tarahumare's blood. Yet
their average life span is about 50 years: They succumb to
disease or infection before circulatory ailments can develop.

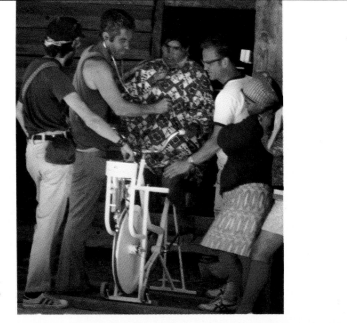

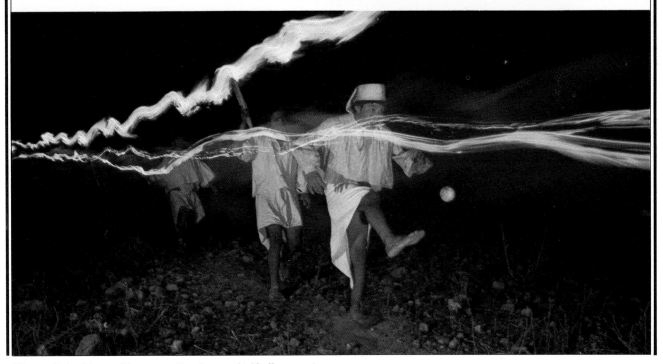

*His way lighted by torchbearers, a Tarahumare kickball racer
punts the wooden sphere. When he tires, one of several teammates
jogging behind will replace him in a rotation that will be
repeated until the race is won, perhaps 72 hours after the start.*

strength 50 to 75 per cent with little or no increase in size. Muscle size, he maintained, depends on the presence of male hormones. Thus female dancers, gymnasts and ice skaters, who need strong muscles to perform their routines, are uniformly slim and feminine looking.

As these facts became more widely known, the attitudes of women toward exercise began to change. In the United States, women joined exercise programs at a faster rate than men; the number of women taking up running in a two-year period went up by 73 per cent; men increased their participation by 53 per cent.

The differences between men and women in their attitudes toward exercise almost disappear as they pass their middle years. Most people in their sixties recognize that they must apply caution in exercise, particularly if they are hindered by heart disease, arthritis or other ailments that seem to accompany old age.

Yet the older a person gets, the more he needs exercise. The heart's ability to pump blood declines about 8 per cent per decade after the twenties. As fatty deposits clog the arteries (a condition known as atherosclerosis), the openings of the coronary arteries narrow—on the average by as much as 30 per cent between the twenties and the fifties. Lung capacity decreases and the chest wall stiffens, so that the amount of oxygen available to body tissues declines. Skeletal muscles, such as the ones in the arms and legs, lose strength; 3 to 5 per cent of the muscle tissue deteriorates each decade. At the same time, fat tissues usually increase. Thus the body's capacity to do work declines by the age of 75 to less than half its capacity at the age of 20. Bones lose calcium, soften, shrink and become more prone to fracture.

Nobody can prevent this deterioration completely, but there is evidence that it can be slowed dramatically by exercise. The counteraging effects of physical activity were demonstrated by researchers at Washington University in St. Louis. They studied a group of men averaging 58 years of age—it included one 72-year-old who had been running regularly for nine years. These men were compared not only with a sedentary group of similar age, but with 10 younger runners averaging 23 years of age. The researchers did not compare the loss of muscle tissue between the two groups of elderly men, but the study did reveal that the lung capacities of the older runners were almost the same as those of the younger athletes and averaged 40 to 50 per cent more than those of the sedentary group. Moreover, the older runners showed only about a 4 per cent decline in work capacity per decade instead of the nearly 8 per cent ordinarily expected.

Other researchers showed that older people who exercise can not only halt the shrinking of bones and even strengthen them but can also slow or stop the deterioration of cartilage in joints that usually comes with age. As Robert E. Wear, Professor of Physical Education at the University of New Hampshire, observed, "People rust out before they wear out because they fail to realize that the human body was made to be used for as long as a person lives."

Convinced of the truth of such assessments, physical therapist Lawrence Frankel, at the request of the West Virginia Commission on Aging, devised in 1970 a set of 50 exercises of varying difficulty and intensity to help old people regain their vigor. The exercises, called Preventicare, were a remarkable success. An early trial at an apartment residence for the elderly in Charleston, West Virginia, involved 15 participants, one of whom, a woman of 75, had become a bedridden invalid. A few weeks after starting Frankel's exercises, the woman was able once again to cook for herself and take care of her apartment. The rejuvenated woman was moved to remark: "Life is worth living again."

Sustaining the effort

Despite the obvious benefits that exercise can confer, some people seem unable to start an active program and continue it regularly. They take exercise as they might a daily dose of medicine—strictly for the benefit they think they will derive. Such a forced approach is almost sure to fail. "There's a high dropout rate," said Dr. Irving Dardik, chairman of the United States Olympic Committee Sports Medicine Council, among people "who rush into a program that is limited to a single activity which is probably something the dropout doesn't truly enjoy anyway. And if he doesn't like to do it, he'll soon find good reasons not to." Professor of

In Cologne, Germany, two gleeful infants float free of their parents' sheltering arms as they paddle underwater in exercise that has been found to aid infant development. Babies can learn to swim at three months; those who start early show better coordination and balance as they grow older than those who first swim at a later age or do not exercise at all.

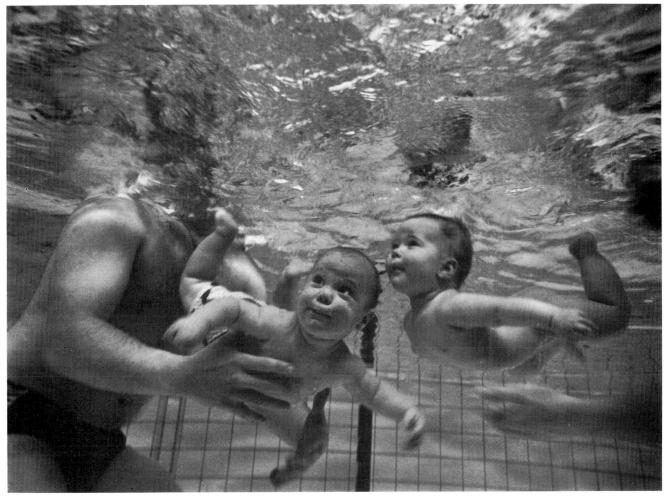

Physical Education Arthur W. Faris of the University of South Alabama in Mobile expressed it differently: "Exercise should be fun."

Exercise can be pleasurable. If you can manage to get through the initial weeks, when the dropout rate is highest, you will probably discover, as millions of others have before you, that you want to continue not because of the uncertain promise of some future benefit, but because regular exercise soon becomes a pleasure and makes you feel good. You will be more relaxed and confident, you will sleep better, and you may even lose weight (and, as a result, become more attractive).

Once you have started exercising regularly, you may be hooked for life. Dr. Gabe Mirkin tells the story of a graduate student in physiology who planned to write his Ph.D. thesis on the effects of discontinuing exercise. He looked for 30 long-term exercisers who would agree to serve as subjects of his experiment by giving up their habit for eight weeks. But he had to abandon the idea; he could not find any exerciser willing to quit. ❋

Working out around the world

Like clothing or cuisine, exercise is part of a people's culture, and the form that physical activity takes is a distinctive mark of national character. Among the people of India, for example, the most popular exercise is hatha-yoga, essentially a discipline emphasizing deep breathing and sinuous postures for relaxation. Though it is thousands of years old, public schools teach it nationwide, and virtually all large Indian cities have yoga instruction centers, either private or government-funded. New Delhi, India's capital, alone supports 25 yoga centers where classes like the one at right are conducted. At the largest of these centers, daily instruction is given to some 1,500 people.

In an ancient culture such as that of India, exercise often carries an added aura of spirituality. So it is with hatha-yoga. Under the tutelage of a guru (the word has the connotation of "teacher" and "spiritual guide"), the serious Indian student of yoga learns the art of mind-clearing meditation and a stringent code of moral behavior, along with specific physical exercises.

Many gurus contend that if a disciple approaches his yogic labors with an attitude of faith and selflessness, he will be rewarded with a treasure of bodily benefits, including freedom from wrinkles, gout, the common cold and sexual impotence. None of these claims have been scientifically proved, but the postures and deep breathing of hatha-yoga undeniably foster flexibility and relaxation—attractions that have drawn a wave of Westerners to yoga classes in recent years.

India is by no means the only country whose people engage in exotic or colorful forms of exercise, as the following pages illustrate. In Japan, assembly lines are halted so that workers can do calisthenics in unison. Scandinavians by the millions carve fields of snow with the tracks of cross-country skis. Strangers assemble in the public squares of China to perform elegant dancelike exercises. And joggers have become as much a symbol of America as instant hamburgers.

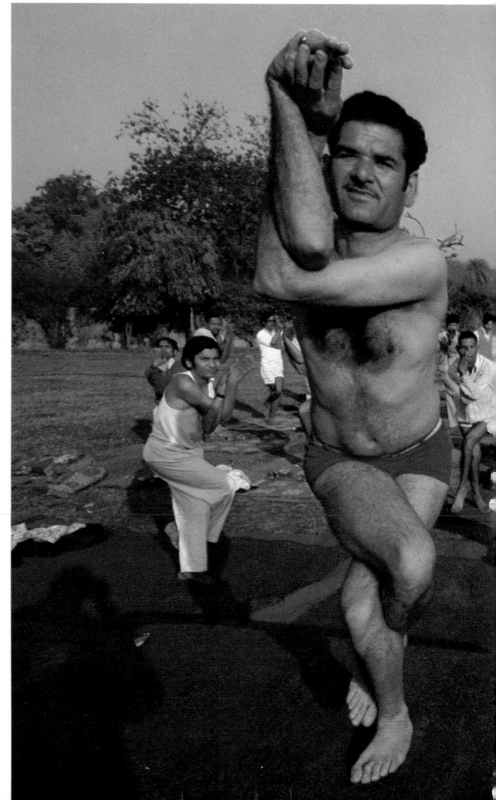

Under the critical eye of their white-robed teacher, members of a New Delhi outdoor yoga class coil their bodies into a posture called the eagle. Among the dozens of yoga exercises, many named for animals, the eagle is considered moderately difficult.

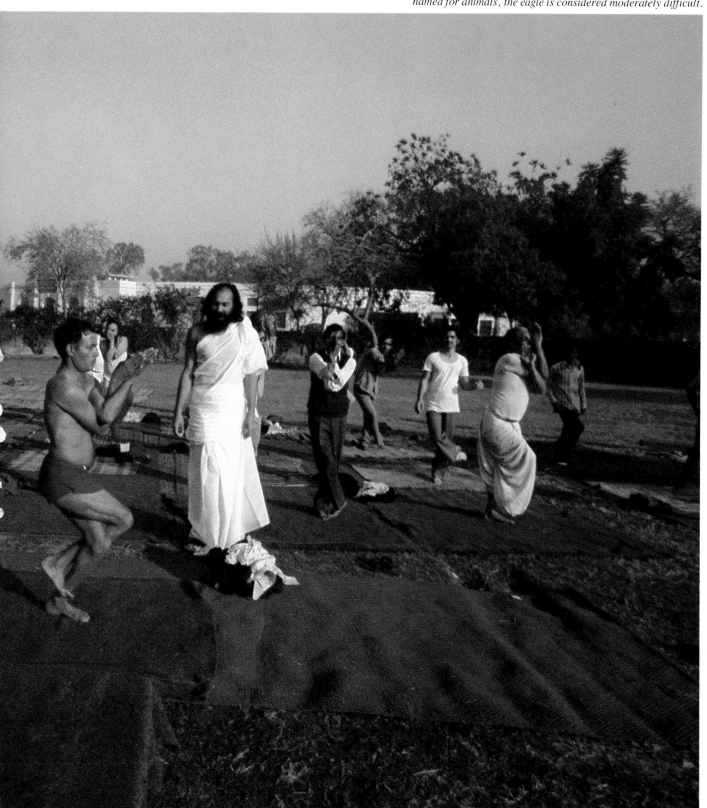

Building a healthier work force in Japan

During an afternoon break at a large Japanese factory, a striking scene unfolds. The clatter of the assembly line is replaced by the blare of martial music from loudspeakers. Workers step from their posts and form an orderly line in the center of the aisle, where, led by one of their fellows, they bend and stretch in time with the music. Five minutes later the calisthenics routine is finished, and work resumes.

Breaks for calisthenics or even brief baseball games are common in Japan—in electronics firms *(right)*, at shipbuilding docks *(opposite)*, in headquarters offices and in government ministries.

Such on-the-job exercises are, in the view of Harvard Professor Edwin O. Reischauer, an authority on Japanese culture, "an expression of the fact that the Japanese like to do things together." In all aspects of Japanese life, Reischauer notes, a premium is placed on group membership and group loyalty, including reciprocal loyalty between employees and employers. Thus Japanese find it natural to join in exercises at their place of work, and employers find it natural, from a paternal concern for the workers' well-being, to provide time and facilities for exercise.

Many businesses sponsor fitness programs far more ambitious than calisthenics breaks. The Osaka Gas Company, for example, spent more than a million dollars on a health services center equipped with a swimming pool, weight room, two tracks for running and an array of other facilities. The center has a full-time staff of 26, including seven doctors to provide checkups and 13 trainers to give periodic physical-fitness evaluations for each of Osaka Gas's 11,500 workers.

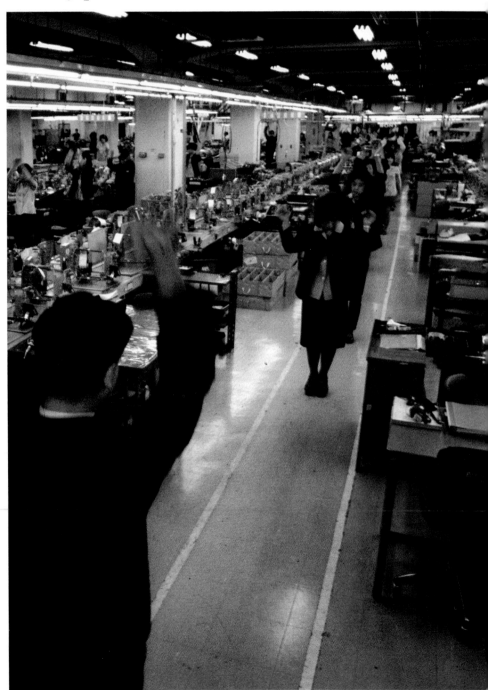

At a Sony television assembly plant in Tokyo, the workday routinely starts off with one of three daily sessions of calisthenics accompanied by martial music; two more five-minute exercise breaks follow at midmorning and after lunch.

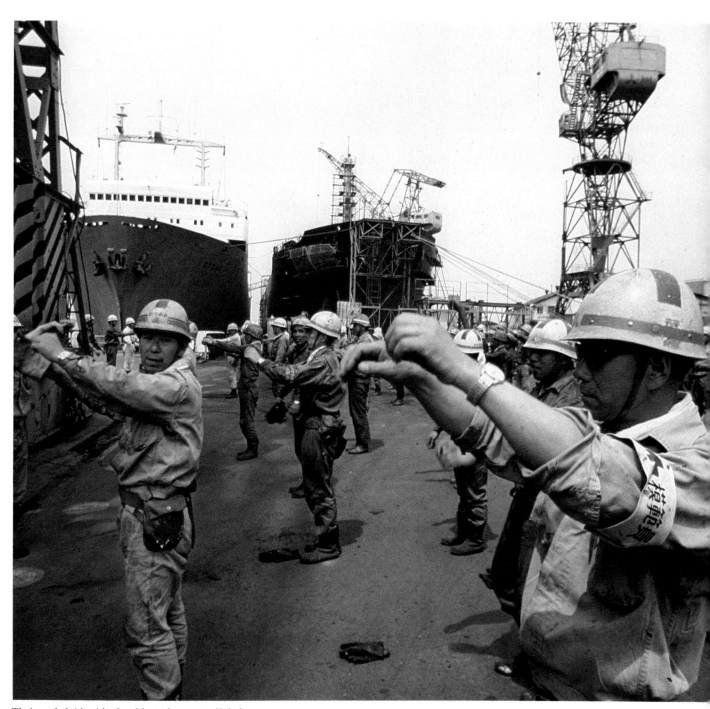

Their tools laid aside, hard-hatted men at a Yokohama shipyard run through their limbering-up exercises. The percentage of Japanese employees participating in such work-break activities more than doubled between 1965 and 1979.

A European tradition of long-distance skiing

A drawing carved on the rock wall of an arctic cave depicts a prehistoric European, skiing on what appear to be long animal bones—testimony to the antiquity of this unique means of travel. Today bone has been replaced by wood and fiberglass, and skiing may no longer be essential as a means of transportation, but it is more popular in the snowy mountains of Europe than ever before—as invigorating winter exercise.

From its origins in Scandinavia—"skiing is the most national of all Norwegian sports," declared arctic explorer Fritdjof Nansen in 1890—this activity has spread across Europe and to other continents. But Norway's low mountains and rolling hills remain its home.

More than one half of Norway's four million citizens ski on cross-country trails. One nationwide association for skiers boasts a membership of 200,000. And every winter weekend, special trains leave Oslo, stopping at points 18¾, 25, 31¼ and 37½ miles away to deposit their passengers—who then ski back to the city along trails that are marked in different colors to denote the degree of difficulty of each route.

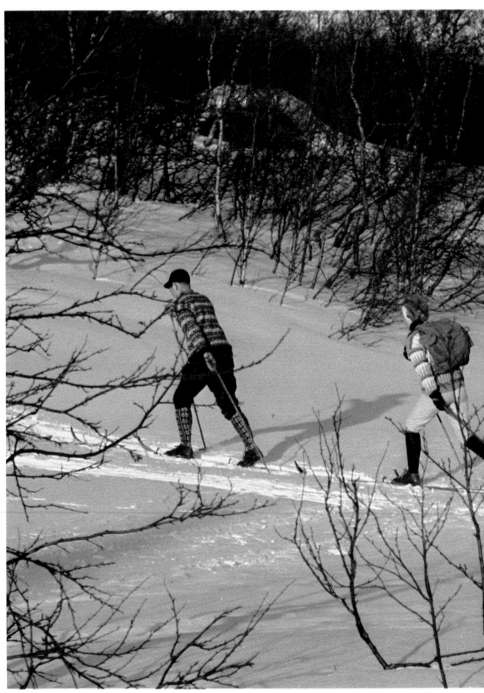

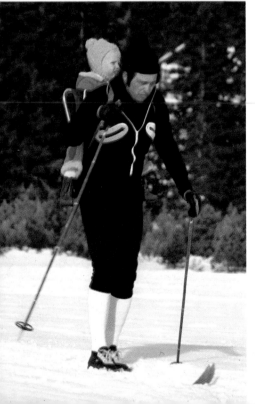

A father carries his son on a ski outing in the foothills of the Alps. In Switzerland, cross-country skiing is a popular form of heart-strengthening aerobic exercise.

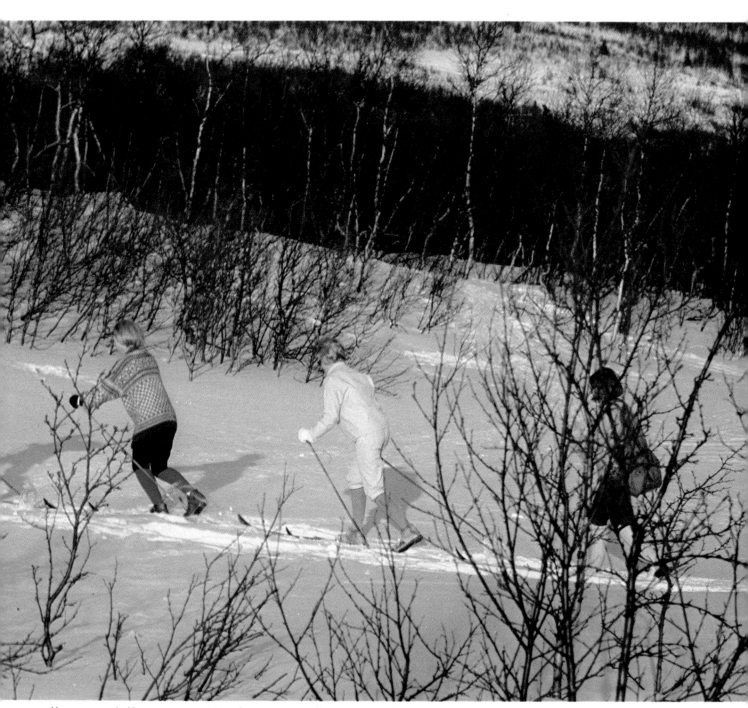

*Near a resort in Norway, a procession of cross-country skiers
ascends a gentle slope. So busy are the trails in that country that
more than 1,000 have been equipped with floodlights for use
after dark—in some cases, around the clock.*

T'ai-chi ch'uan: an ancient ritual of dancelike grace

Masters of the Chinese exercise called *t'ai-chi ch'uan,* or simply *t'ai-chi,* often think of it in poetic terms. One teacher compares it to "swimming in air." Others ask their students to imagine that they are marionettes, or that their torsos are trees.

Such notions come easily to mind at the sight of the slow, stylized *t'ai-chi* movements. Millions of Chinese practice the 128 postures at dawn and dusk each day. Because the postures usually follow the same order, strangers can meet to perform all or part of them in unison, as though they had been rehearsing together for weeks.

Throughout a typical 20-minute round of *t'ai-chi* the spine remains straight; the arms and legs are in constant motion. *T'ai-chi* requires neither the contortions of yoga nor the exertions of Western exercise. "*T'ai-chi* is based on effortlessness," wrote one teacher. "All unnecessary exertion is avoided."

Oddly, this gentle exercise is also a form of self-defense: The words *t'ai-chi ch'uan* mean "supreme ultimate boxing." *T'ai-chi* uses not brute strength but leverage. By leaning away from an attack, a master can throw an assailant off balance, making him vulnerable.

T'ai-chi has been traced at least as far back as the Sung Dynasty (960-1278 A.D.), and it is bound up in much older systems of philosophy. Modern adherents still claim for it a wide range of curative powers. But even those who disdain its metaphysical trappings welcome its ability to limber the body, relax tensions and promote circulation.

In Shanghai a six-year-old begins her day with a round of exercise that is a prelude to t'ai-chi ch'uan. The postures of t'ai-chi are performed by old and young alike.

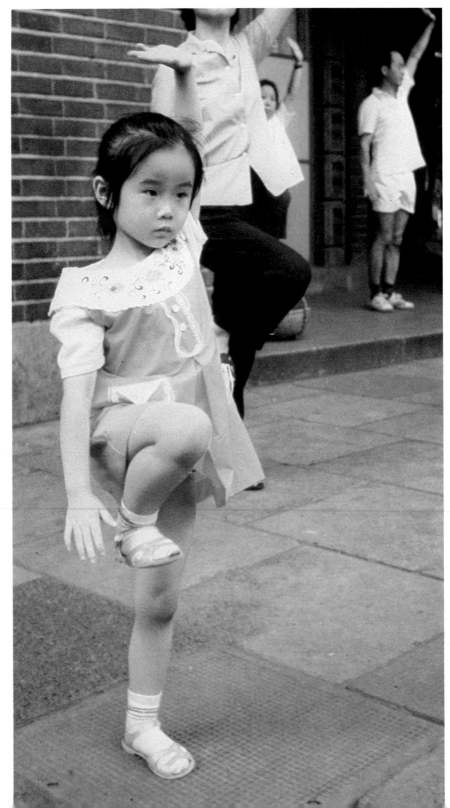

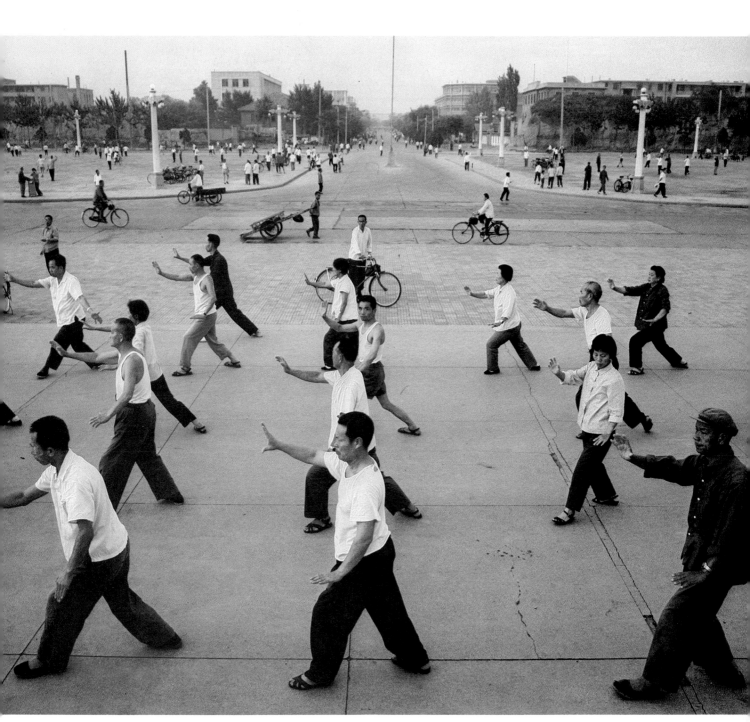

*An impromptu t'ai-chi ch'uan class runs through its paces
as dawn lights the main square of a Chinese town. T'ai-chi can
be practiced anywhere, and is a common sight whenever people
have a few minutes free—waiting at bus stops, for instance.*

In America, a passion for jogging

As recently as the mid-1960s a man jogging through his neighborhood in Hartford, Connecticut, was headed off by a police car and handed a ticket for illegal use of a highway. Legally guilty or not, that runner was moving in the right direction, for jogging is a beneficially strenuous exercise that aids the circulatory and respiratory systems. And in the United States it has become the most common of all the activities spawned by the fitness boom of the 1960s and 1970s.

By the end of the 1970s, some 17 million Americans ran regularly, and in a poll of Washington, D.C., residents, 23 per cent of the respondents claimed to be frequent runners—a higher percentage than took part in any other exercise. Magazines edited especially for runners rate jogging shoes, offer tips to combat fatigue or injury and list upcoming running events from Land O'Lakes, Florida, to Puyallup, Washington. Running, concluded one American writer, "is as much a part of our culture as blue jeans."

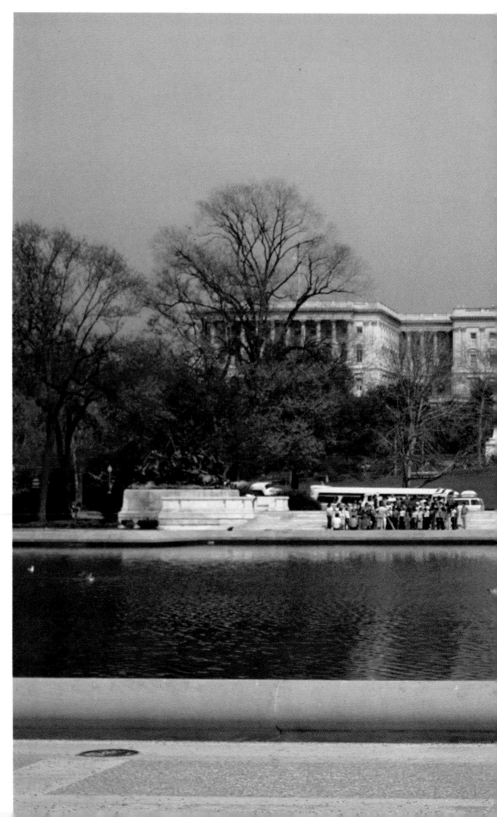

A pair of brightly clad joggers trot past the Reflecting Pool below the United States Capitol in Washington, D.C., where almost 20 miles of specially constructed trails provide for traffic-free running.

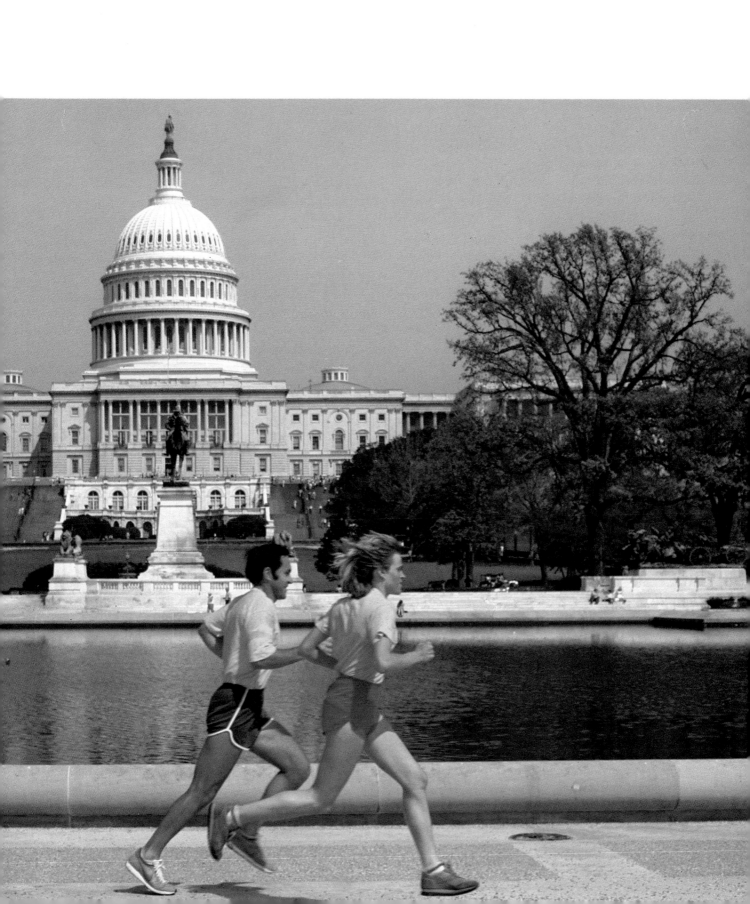

CHAPTER 2

What exercise can do for you

A prescription for stamina
Brawn for everyday tasks
Taking off flab
Supple muscles, limber joints
Balm for frazzled nerves

It is midday at a health club in Paris. Dozens of men strain to lift weights, do push-ups and sit-ups, and manipulate exercise machines. In a room nearby, a group of men and women are practicing yoga.

An hour before daybreak in a fashionable neighborhood of Dallas, two dozen middle-aged men outfitted in shorts and T-shirts run off together into the darkness. Halfway around the world, hundreds of Japanese men and women jog alongside the moat of the Imperial Palace in Tokyo.

Every day, in Geneva and Paris, New York and San Francisco, Manila and Peking, millions of people spend hours running, bicycling, rope jumping, weight lifting, playing tennis or football, walking, swimming or shadow boxing. There are scores of such exercises, and the physical effects of one differ subtly from the effects of any other. Yet the variety of exercises is less confusing and diverse than it seems. Each leads to at least one of five fitness goals: greater stamina from a strengthened heart and circulatory system; increased power in the muscles; a trimmer and slimmer body; greater flexibility and joint mobility; and relaxation of tensions. Of all these goals the most important, say fitness experts, is a strengthened circulatory system.

Many exercises promote several of these goals simultaneously. Jogging, cycling and swimming not only improve heart action and stamina but also strengthen certain muscles. Calisthenics build strength and flexibility—and can help the heart if they involve running in place or similar continuous activity. Sports may develop stamina, strength and flexibility

(or they may help not at all, depending on what game is played and how hard and long it is played). Yoga can be done for relaxation, but it improves flexibility as well. And almost all exercises have some effect on the shape of the body.

Which goals you choose to pursue are up to you. So are the means of achieving them. There is no compelling reason to limit yourself to one goal or to work toward all five. Some people concentrate on one activity. Others select a varied exercise menu. Either approach can produce good results.

Until the early 1960s, few physicians—and fewer nonprofessionals—knew just how much exercise was good or necessary. Some doctors actively discouraged exercise. For example, in the early 1950s, Dr. Peter Steincrohn in a book entitled *How to Keep Fit Without Exercise* not only asserted "exercise is bosh" but concluded "to have a strong heart it is essential to give up all unnecessary exercise." Most people thought, however, that exercise was probably a good idea, yet anyone who asked a doctor about it was almost always told to go ahead, with a warning: "Don't overdo it." Beyond that vague caution, specific guidelines were seldom offered.

In 1961, a young United States Air Force doctor, Captain Kenneth Cooper, began experimenting to find what kind of exercise would be best for the astronauts who were then being trained for the Manned Orbiting Laboratory project, planned for the late 1960s. Although his interest lay with the astronauts, his subjects also included thousands of airmen in all kinds of jobs and in all kinds of physical condition—from flabby and overweight to trim and muscular.

Norman Rockwell portrayed the timeless interest in the benefits of exercise in this picture of a spindly young weight lifter that he painted for a magazine cover in 1922.

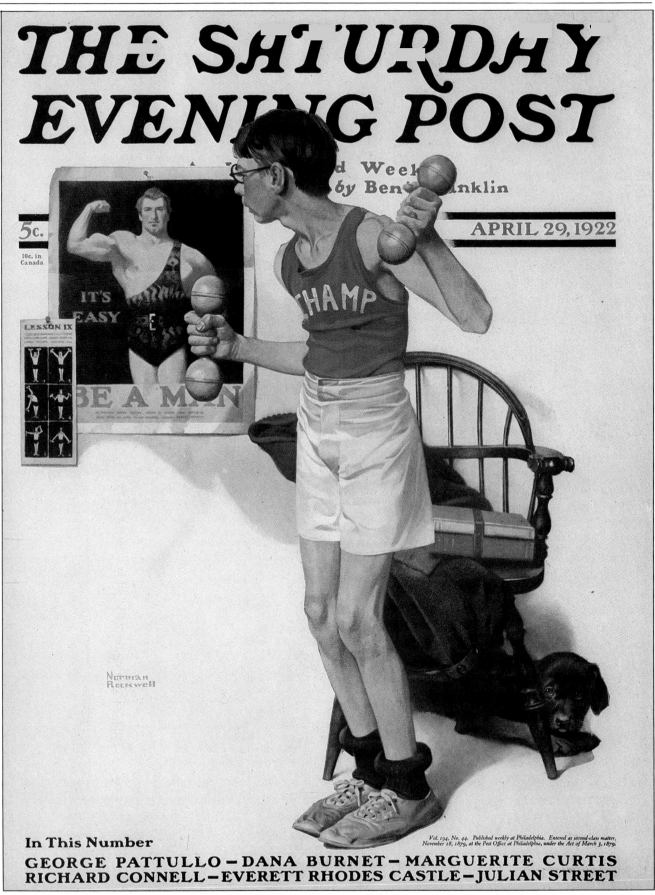

THE SATURDAY EVENING POST

APRIL 29, 1922

In This Number

GEORGE PATTULLO — DANA BURNET — MARGUERITE CURTIS
RICHARD CONNELL — EVERETT RHODES CASTLE — JULIAN STREET

Dr. Cooper had at his disposal complicated laboratory equipment, which he used to gauge the capacities of his subjects' bodies. He checked the size and strength of their muscles. He took their pulse rates and calculated the ratio of lean muscle to fat in their bodies. He measured how much air their lungs could take in and expel and even how much blood each heartbeat pumped into their arteries through their bodies. To test endurance, he put the men on treadmills and made them run until they were exhausted.

Dr. Cooper found that the men who lasted longest on the treadmill did not have exceptionally strong muscles. But they were also not overweight, and the proportion of fat to lean muscle in their bodies was low. At rest, they had lower pulse rates than the subjects who became exhausted most rapidly on the treadmill, in part because their hearts pumped nearly twice as much blood with each beat. And the lungs of the men with great endurance could take in and expel one and one half times as much air as those of the more easily tired subjects.

Then Dr. Cooper analyzed the gases exhaled by the airmen as they ran on the treadmill. Those who excelled at this test had a higher oxygen consumption than the others, a measurement that is called by physiologists VO_2max—"V" for volume, "O_2" for oxygen in the air and "max" for maximum.

VO_2max is the volume of oxygen that the body uses up when it is working as hard as it can. This factor indicates how efficiently the body can make use of oxygen because, in order to perform work like that of exercising on a treadmill, muscles must produce energy, a process in which oxygen plays an important role. Greater oxygen consumption is thus a sign of greater capacity for energy production and work— greater endurance. People with a high VO_2max can do much more work before tiring than those with a low VO_2max.

Up to this point, Dr. Cooper's work covered ground that had already been explored on a smaller scale elsewhere in the United States and in Europe. As early as the 1930s, researchers had tried to learn what happens to the human body when it is exercising. The earliest studies, conducted in Germany and Scandinavia, dealt with the circulatory system. Researchers investigated how the heart pumps blood during exercise and how the body apportions the blood flow be-

tween exercising muscles and other organs under less strain. In the mid-1950s, physiologists at the University of Minnesota suggested that the body's ability to use oxygen might be a reliable indicator of the capacities of the circulatory and respiratory systems.

These experiments laid the foundation for establishing a relationship between endurance, as measured by a test on a treadmill or a stationary bicycle, and several characteristics generally accepted as marks of physical fitness: low pulse rate, lean body, high blood-pumping rate and high breathing capacity. Then Dr. Cooper went a step further. He hypothesized that one measurement—VO_2max, the proficiency with which the body extracts oxygen from breathed air and delivers it to the muscles—served to assess this relationship. And because VO_2max depends on the performance of two of the body's most important systems—the circulatory and the respiratory—Dr. Cooper concluded that VO_2max is a measure of basic fitness: People with a high VO_2max are fit; those with a lower VO_2max are not.

From his observations and tests, he was able to determine a specific value for the minimum VO_2max required for good

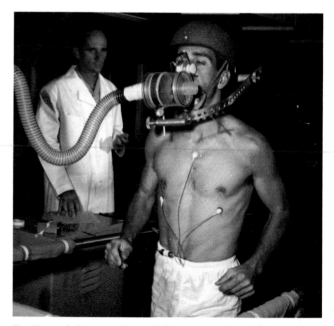

Dr. Kenneth Cooper, whose Air Force research and later writings helped set off the 1970s boom in exercise, observes a fellow officer during a treadmill test in 1968. The large plastic cylinder, supported by a metal strap attached to the GI helmet liner, is used to collect exhaled breath from the subject in order to measure his oxygen consumption.

physical condition. Subjects who could be considered fit (judging by such characteristics as pulse rate, fat content and performance on the treadmill) had a VO₂max of at least 42 milliliters of oxygen consumed per minute per kilogram of body weight (1.16 cubic inches per minute per pound). Though this figure is greater than the 21-to-37-milliliter VO₂max, depending on age and sex, for the sedentary individual, it is small in comparison to a highly trained athlete's rate of oxygen consumption. The VO₂maxes of the world's top long-distance runners range from 70 milliliters to well above 80 milliliters per minute per kilogram. Even the VO₂max of healthy slugs has now been measured. Mark Denny of the University of British Columbia in Vancouver found it to be about half a milliliter per minute per kilogram for the slugs' top speed of about one inch per minute.

Slugs and world-class athletes aside, it seemed to Dr. Cooper that those with a VO₂max of 42 or better—slightly less if they were more than 35 years old—were able to pursue their everyday activities with their bodies in effect running at idle, while those with a lower VO₂max raced their biological engines through life, a practice that Dr. Cooper felt could wear them out prematurely.

The results of Dr. Cooper's experiments repeated themselves so consistently that he became adept at predicting a new subject's endurance and VO₂max simply by asking questions about his physical activities. Men who took frequent long walks, rode a bicycle to work or swam regularly always performed better on the treadmill test than men who did no exercise; surprisingly, they also did better than men who played golf, tennis doubles or other sports that most people had always thought of as good exercise. They even did better than muscular specimens who devoted themselves to daily regimens of calisthenics or exercise with weights, widely presumed to be the kinds of exercise that contribute most to overall fitness and good health.

It became evident to Dr. Cooper that anyone who wished to experience the benefits of a high VO₂max could do so simply by taking up walking, running or some other activity associated with endurance on the treadmill test. To get the biological engine running at idle most of the time, Dr. Coo-

per suggested, its owner had to speed it up regularly. These endurance exercises he called aerobics (from a word meaning ''in the presence of oxygen''), to express the biochemical connection between the exercises and VO₂max.

To make it easy to keep track of increases in oxygen consumption, Dr. Cooper devised a system of points based on results of his experiments. He found that anyone who ran one mile in less than eight minutes six times a week could pass the treadmill test with a VO₂max of at least 42 cubic centimeters of oxygen per minute per kilogram, his definition of a good level of physical fitness.

Dr. Cooper arbitrarily assigned a value of 30 points, or five points for each of the six eight-minute miles, to this ration of exercise. Then, using a variety of methods, he compared the oxygen consumptions of men running faster and slower—as well as of men engaged in other exercises and sports—and assigned points accordingly. Running four miles in 40 minutes, for example, was worth 12 points. Cycling 10 miles in less than half an hour earned 15 points. A 20-minute game of handball counted three points.

After four years' research, Dr. Cooper compiled his re-

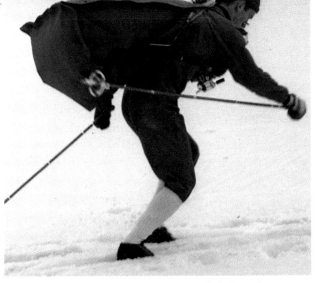

A cross-country skier exhales into a sack called a Douglas bag (named for its British inventor, Dr. Claude Gordon Douglas). Chemical analysis of gases collected in this way indicates that skiers and other athletes engaged in strenuous exercise can, with conditioning, increase by 20 per cent or more the rate at which their bodies use oxygen to make energy—a key measure of fitness.

sults into detailed tables, which allowed an exerciser to select combinations of activities that added up to 30 points per week—enough exercise, the running experiments had shown, to produce fitness and maintain it. Using this rather complex system of points, Dr. Cooper was able to give more specific advice than "don't overdo it" about how much of what kind of exercise is good for health.

Dr. Cooper surprised many people when he declared that calisthenics, weight lifting and other favorite exercises, while fine for certain purposes, were essentially useless in building VO2max. But in the years that followed, his findings were duplicated and confirmed in other laboratories. Though physiologists have refined his conclusions—they have devised a method for gauging exercise *(Chapter 3)* that compensates for small variations in the intensity of exercise as well as hills and head winds—no one disputes Dr. Cooper's hypothesis that physical fitness is best measured by oxygen consumption. For anyone who wants to get in shape, then, aerobic exercise that increases VO2max is essential, although other types of activity may be needed to limber the body, to relax tensions, to provide a more attractive shape or to build strength.

A prescription for stamina

Most physiologists believe that aerobic exercises make for healthier hearts and circulatory systems because of what is called the overload principle, which has been demonstrated repeatedly in the laboratory.

Overloading a set of muscles—exercising them at a level above which they normally operate—obviously will tire them. But the laboratory experiments showed that when muscles that have been tired by overloading have had time to recover, they reset themselves to a slightly higher potential. The process repeats if the strengthened muscles are again stressed to this limit. A system of exercise that alternates overload and rest in this way takes muscles to remarkable levels of strength and endurance. The process has led to a world record for continuous swimming of 168 hours—a solid week, night and day. For nonstop walking, the record is 148 hours 31 minutes over a distance of 317 miles. A man once hiked cross-country, 32 miles a day for 81 consecutive weeks, covering a distance of more than 18,000 miles. Such stamina is of course superfluous for everyday living, but the process that produced it can help ordinary people achieve a healthy level of endurance.

The most valuable effect of overloading is believed to be on the heart. Aerobic exercise presumably forces the heart to beat faster than usual to pump the more-than-normal amount of oxygen-rich blood needed by the muscles being exercised. As the heart recuperates between exercise sessions, it becomes slightly stronger and does not have to work quite so hard the next time to satisfy the demands of the muscles.

The effect on the heart has been confirmed in animals through autopsy; aerobic exercise does increase the size of their hearts and blood vessels. In humans, increases in heart size have been detected with a kind of medical sonar that bounces high-pitched sound waves off the heart to make it visible. A study of athletes by the United States National Institutes of Health showed that runners and swimmers had hearts that weighed almost 50 per cent more than those of people of the same ages and sex who were not regular participants in sports. This sound-wave technique does not show blood vessels and there is no conclusive evidence that human blood vessels become larger with exercise. But it is known that after several months of exercise, humans' heart rates and blood pressures decrease while endurance increases, and it is also known that such changes are an indication of a larger, stronger heart and blood vessels.

The overload principle works on the lungs as well. Aerobic exercise forces them to take in and expel more air than usual. As a result, chest muscles and the diaphragm—the dome-shaped sheet of muscle below the lungs that causes air to rush in and out of them—are worked harder than usual. Like the heart, these muscles presumably become stronger between exercise sessions and breathing becomes progressively less labored. Other muscles that are exercised become stronger, so that walking, bicycle riding or swimming can be continued longer without fatigue.

Collectively, all these bodily changes are referred to as the training effect, and in people who exercise regularly it can

A three-minute test of stamina

Using the simple "step test" illustrated at right, you can rate the ability of your heart and lungs to supply your body with oxygen—your aerobic fitness—which serves as a measure of stamina and all-around physical condition. The test gauges oxygen use by indicating how much your heartbeat slows down after it has been forced to speed up. A quick recovery toward a slow heartbeat is considered by physiologists to be a sign of fitness.

For this test, you need a stopwatch and a sturdy platform, exactly eight inches high, to serve as a step—a cinder block, for example. Because you must step at a constant tempo, a metronome set at 96 is helpful; however, a friend calling out the rhythm, or your own careful eye on the stopwatch, will serve equally well to keep you stepping in time.

To take the test, you must step on and off the platform 72 times in three minutes (right, top), pause 30 seconds, then count your heartbeats (right, bottom) for 30 seconds. The table below converts the number of beats into a level of aerobic fitness. For most people, this test is not too strenuous. But if while taking it you experience shortness of breath, dizziness or any pain, stop at once. Consult your doctor before trying again or exercising.

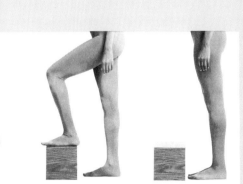

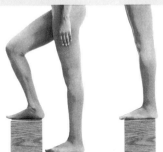

UP AND DOWN, 24 TIMES A MINUTE
Four motions make up the step test. Step up first with one foot (1), then with the other (2). Next, step down with the first foot (3) and then with the second (4). Repeat the cycle once every 2½ seconds (if you have a metronome, move one foot at every beat). After three minutes of stepping, sit down and rest for 30 seconds without talking.

COUNTING YOUR HEARTBEATS
After resting 30 seconds, lightly place three finger tips on your neck, just beneath your jawbone and to one side of your Adam's apple. Using the stopwatch, count for 30 seconds the number of throbs you feel in the large artery under your finger tips.

CONVERTING HEARTBEAT TO FITNESS LEVEL
To use the table at right, find in the column of figures that applies to your age and sex the number of heartbeats that you counted—30 seconds' worth, beginning 30 seconds after the step test. Then read your level of aerobic fitness at the left of the table. For example, if you are a 45-year-old man and counted 52 heartbeats, you fall into the "fair" range of fitness.

Heartbeat Count after Step Test

FITNESS	Age 20-29		Age 30-39		Age 40-49		Age 50 and over	
	MEN	WOMEN	MEN	WOMEN	MEN	WOMEN	MEN	WOMEN
Excellent	37 or less	43 or less	39 or less	43 or less	40 or less	44 or less	41 or less	45 or less
Good	38-42	44-46	40-43	44-47	41-44	45-47	42-45	46-49
Fair	43-50	47-55	44-50	48-56	45-52	48-57	46-52	50-58
Poor	51 or more	56 or more	51 or more	57 or more	53 or more	58 or more	53 or more	59 or more

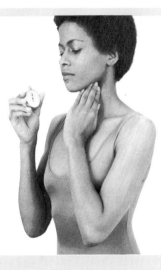

cause astounding improvements in just a few months, as Dr. Cooper proved time and again with members of the Air Force. As one example—and not an altogether unusual one—of what physical activity can accomplish, Dr. Norbert Sander of The Preventive & Sports Medicine Center in New York City told of a patient whose blood pressure was dangerously high. On the treadmill test he performed poorly, lasting only seven minutes before he was too exhausted to continue.

The test results left Dr. Sander no choice but to prescribe only the mildest form of aerobic exercise—slow walking and riding a stationary bicycle—to improve the patient's fitness. But as his aerobic capacities improved, the length of time he exercised was increased, until after six months he could walk three miles six days a week. On three of those days, he also cycled for 30 minutes. Dr. Sander reexamined him at this point. Though aerobic exercise cannot be counted on to cure hypertension, this man's blood pressure had dropped into the normal range, and his pulse rate at rest had decreased from 104 beats per minute to 80. On the treadmill he more than doubled his endurance, bringing it to a level that was average for a man of his age.

Part of the reason treadmill performance improved is that aerobic exercise builds muscles other than heart muscle— the ones in the legs are helped by walking, running or bicycling, those in the chest by swimming—while it increases stamina. This new strength allows exercise at a higher level—more strenuous and more prolonged—before fatigue sets in. But building up the heart, not improving strength, is the main purpose of aerobic exercises. For greater strength, aerobic exercises must be supplemented with others.

Brawn for everyday tasks

Ideally, between one quarter and one half of body weight should be muscle. There are three types. One is in the heart. Another consists of the muscles that move food through the digestive tract. Skeletal muscles constitute the third type; there are more than 400 of these, attached to the bones by tendons, and together they control the body's movements.

If the skeletal muscles are weak, they hinder the routine lifting and carrying that are a part of everyone's life. More important, weak muscles are easily overloaded to the point of injury, so that a heavy box can be a painful hazard if lifted with muscles that are not strong enough for the job. Indeed, chronic pain in the lower back, a common complaint, may be caused by weak muscles in the abdomen; these often help allow a paunch to develop—a constant load that the back muscles must support.

In any sport muscular strength is obviously essential; superior strength can help anyone excel. Some tennis players, to increase the speed of their strokes, use a dumbbell that weighs up to 10 times as much as a racket. Baseball players swing a weighted bat to improve their power at the plate.

In strengthening skeletal muscles, as in strengthening the heart, the overload principle is at work. A muscle becomes stronger when it must work harder than it has been accus-

---

An antidote for cigarettes?

According to conventional wisdom, exercise offers an antidote for the cigarette habit. But a Harris poll showed that conventional wisdom is wrong. Americans who exercised were about as likely to smoke as those who did not.

More surprising were comparisons between different exercisers. Those who were most active (men and women who averaged five or more hours of exercise per week) included about the same percentage of smokers as the least active group (averaging two and a half or fewer hours per week). Moderate exercisers, however, included 12 per cent fewer smokers than the other two groups.

The kind of exercise performed made even more difference than the amount. Cigarettes were smoked by 45 per cent of the swimmers and 41 per cent of those who did calisthenics—but by only 24 per cent of the runners, 30 per cent of walkers and 28 per cent of participants in racket sports such as tennis. The lesson seems clear: Someone who exercises moderately—roughly, three to four hours a week—at such activities as running, walking and racket sports is least likely to be a cigarette smoker. But it is clear only up to a point. No one can say the connection is not coincidence—and there is no proof that exercise helps to kick the cigarette habit.

tomed to, and then rests. As it rests, it resets itself at a slightly higher level of performance. What was once difficult becomes easier, and the load can be increased again. In this way strength improves dramatically.

There are two types of exercise that are used to develop strength in the muscles. They are isometrics, in which the muscles remain stationary, and isotonics, in which they move. (A third kind of strength-building exercise, called isokinetic training, is unavailable to most people. The equipment it requires is expensive and so complicated to use properly that a specially trained person is needed to set it up correctly. It is used mainly for physical therapy to rebuild muscle injured in accidents or on the playing field.)

In isometric training, a muscle's force is pitted against an immovable object. You can stand in a doorway, for example, and try to push opposite sides apart, or you can hook your finger tips together and pull outward vigorously. Little or no movement occurs, but the muscle develops considerable force by exerting effort against the resistance.

This form of exercise had a flurry of popularity in the 1950s and 1960s. German exercise physiologists demonstrated that an exerciser who performed a single maximum contraction of a muscle for one second a day would increase the muscle's strength by an astonishing 5 per cent a week. But later research revealed that isometric training has a severe limitation. A muscle strengthened by one kind of exertion is not necessarily strengthened for a different exertion. Strength is increased at the angle made by arm or leg joints when the exercise is performed, but not at other joint angles. When you stand in a doorway and press against its sides, your elbow, wrist and shoulder joints are set at very specific angles that depend on the size of your frame and the size of the doorframe. Your muscles are strengthened almost entirely for pushing at those angles and no others; your ability to lift a box, for example, will be little improved because the joint angles for that effort are different from the joint angles for the isometric exercise.

Thus to train a muscle throughout its range of motion, and not at just one specific position, a person would have to go through a series of isometric exercises, each one performed

One of the most famous of all promotions is the "97-pound weakling" advertisement by Charles Atlas for his Dynamic-Tension body-building program. Appearing in eight languages over more than 50 years, it touted isometric exercises as a better way of "making a man out of 'Mac'" than the weight lifting that inspired Norman Rockwell's painting on page 35.

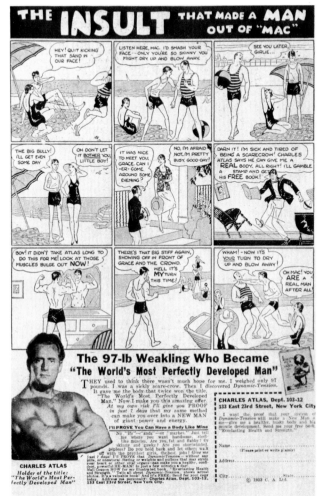

in a slightly different position for each muscle. So in recent years isometric training has been used largely by physical therapists in the rehabilitation of muscles that have a small, well-defined area of weakness.

Isometric exercises have gone out of favor for another reason: They can be dangerous. Applying maximum force during isometric exercises usually closes the glottis, the narrowest part of the windpipe, between the vocal cords. A closed glottis prevents exhalation. Thus as the muscles (in-

To test the strength of every muscle

Because muscular strength varies greatly from one part of the body to another, tests of strength require devices such as those at the University of Denver Human Performance Laboratory *(below)*, which measure one muscle group at a time. One machine can even gauge the strength of the muscles that move a thumb. The laboratory devices are called tensiometers. They measure the tension (in pounds) generated on a spring-loaded plunger by a cable strapped to the subject. The strength of some 38 different muscle groups can be gauged in this way. For many of the tests, parts of the subject's body must be forcibly held stationary by a technician *(below, right)* so that only one muscle group—the group being gauged—is able to pull against the plunger.

Although laboratory equipment is needed for accurate strength measurements, a rough idea of the strength of certain muscle groups is provided by simple tests. The YMCA, for example, evaluates the strength of stomach muscles of participants in its exercise classes by counting the number of sit-ups that they can complete in one minute. The average man under 35 years of age performs 33, the average woman 25; the scores for those over 35 are 27 and 18 respectively.

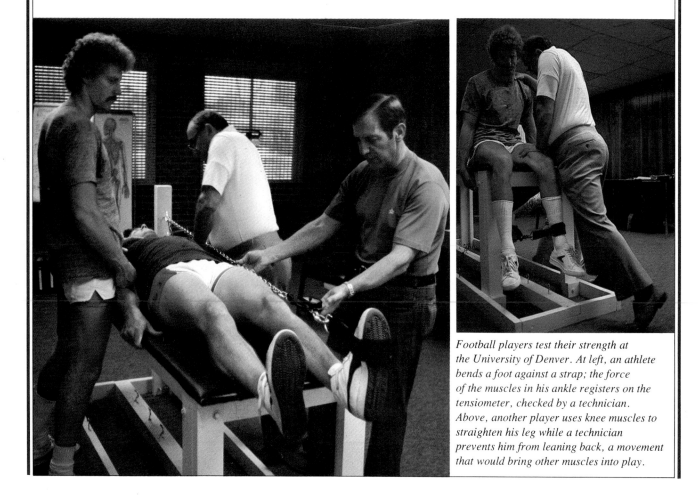

Football players test their strength at the University of Denver. At left, an athlete bends a foot against a strap; the force of the muscles in his ankle registers on the tensiometer, checked by a technician. Above, another player uses knee muscles to straighten his leg while a technician prevents him from leaning back, a movement that would bring other muscles into play.

cluding those of the chest) contract vigorously, the pressure in the lungs rises sharply. This pressure travels through the thin walls of the lungs to the veins in the chest region. The pressure compresses the veins and reduces blood flow into the heart and to the brain; the reduction in blood flow may cause dizziness, spots before the eyes or even fainting.

Perhaps more serious, the contraction of muscles in isometric exercises greatly increases their resistance to blood flow. This causes a sharp rise in blood pressure and a consequent increase in the work load of the heart. For this reason, people with heart or blood-vessel disease should not perform isometric exercises. Even those without this ailment conceivably could harm themselves with isometrics. Fatal brain hemorrhages have been induced not by exercise but by strain similar to that caused by isometric exertion—in some instances trying too hard to move too heavy a box has burst blood vessels in the brain. Better and safer for everyone are rhythmic isotonic exercises, which promote steady blood flow and result in little increase in blood pressure.

In isotonic exercises the muscles move a weight through their entire range of motion. Virtually any object can be adapted as a weight for isotonic exercises. (It should never be so heavy that you must push with all your might to move it; the exercise would then pose the same dangers as an isometric one.) Calisthenics such as push-ups and pull-ups, for example, use the weight of the entire body to strengthen the arm, chest and back muscles. The same results can be achieved by lifting books or bags of sand. However, most people who exercise with weights reject such makeshift apparatus in favor of barbells and dumbbells.

Women traditionally have shunned these kinds of activity. Even today, when athletic prowess is no longer considered irreconcilable with femininity, women are reluctant to take up strength-building exercises because they do not want to develop prominent muscles. Yet stronger arm, chest and back muscles could substantially ease the carrying and lifting that women do every day, to say nothing of improving their games of tennis and golf.

For the majority of women the fear of becoming over-muscled has been proved groundless by the experiments of Jack Wilmore, Professor of Physical Education at the University of Arizona. Wilmore put male and female student volunteers through a 10-week exercise regimen to compare the effects of identical exercises on men's and women's strength and physiques.

The men, as expected, were able to lift heavier weights than the women, both before and after the experiments. However, when the results were adjusted for the differences between the sexes in the total amount of muscle tissue, male superiority disappeared. Ounce for ounce of muscle, the women were as strong as the men. Furthermore, the training exercises caused almost no change in the size of the women's muscles. One of the largest increases in muscle girth was measured on the women's upper arms at the biceps; they grew an average of only about a quarter inch. Yet the women's strength improved by 11 to 30 per cent, depending on the exercise. The men's muscles grew up to five times as much as the women's muscles but had no greater gains in relative strength. Wilmore concluded that larger muscles are ''not a necessary consequence of gains in strength.''

It is true that some female body builders possess muscles that grow substantially when they work out several hours a day. Scientists have not yet determined why some women develop bulging muscles and others, no matter how hard they exercise, do not. The only way a woman can find out whether her muscles are the kind that grow is to try exercising. If the muscles get too big, stopping the exercise will quickly cause them to shrink to their former size.

The explanation for the difference between men and women in their tendency to become more muscular with exercise probably lies in the amount of testosterone, the principal male hormone, in the body. Experiments conducted by Dr. Theodor Hettinger during the 1950s in Dortmund, Germany, showed that men who had extra testosterone injected into their bodies became muscular faster than men who did not receive the hormone shots. Dr. Hettinger did not perform the same experiment on women; if he had, he might have conclusively demonstrated the role of testosterone. Nevertheless, it is widely thought that women run little risk of creating unsightly bulges of muscle, because they com-

Finding out how much of you is fat

The bathroom scale is an untrustworthy instrument for measuring how fat you are—the tables that relate weight to overweight are crude. But an easy-to-use home procedure for gauging your percentage of body fat requires only three body measurements, made with a cloth tape, and four arithmetic steps, performed with the aid of the tables at right. In following the procedures, choose the color-coded figure that represents your age and sex. Measure the part of the body indicated on the appropriate figure for each step. Look up that measurement in the adjoining table. The places to measure, indicated by black lines on the figures, are shown more accurately on large drawings at right.

The measurements and tables provide four separate numbers, one in each step, that are combined as indicated by the boxes at the bottom of the opposite page to compute the percentage of body fat. A percentage above 15 per cent for men or more than 25 per cent for women is considered a health hazard and should be reduced by exercise and diet.

To check progress in losing fat, repeat these procedures every three weeks.

WHERE TO MEASURE

The locations of the measurements for the test on the opposite page are indicated directly on the drawings at right. Measure your forearm, buttocks and calf where those features are largest in circumference; measure your abdomen one half inch above your navel, your thigh just below the curve of your buttocks, and your upper arm at a point midway between shoulder and elbow. Be sure that the tape is not pulled so tight that it depresses the skin and thus distorts the measurement.

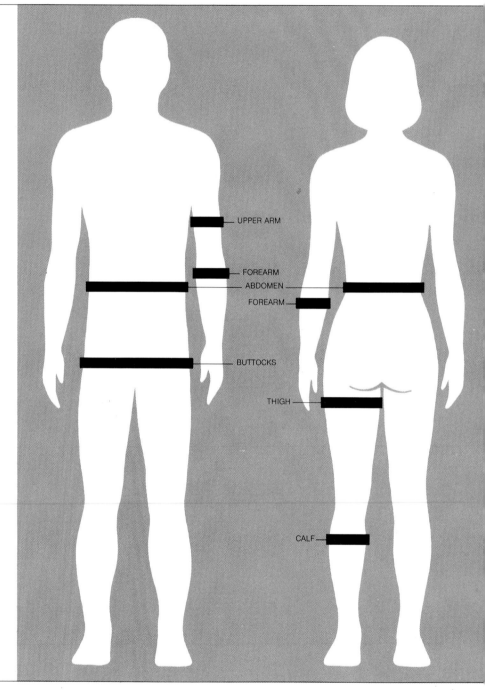

UPPER ARM

FOREARM

ABDOMEN

FOREARM

BUTTOCKS

THIGH

CALF

| WOMEN 35 AND YOUNGER |
| WOMEN 36 AND OLDER |
| MEN 35 AND YOUNGER |
| MEN 36 AND OLDER |

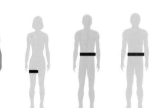

STEP 1: *Find the drawing (left) for your sex and age, then measure to the nearest inch the circumference of your body as indicated by the black line on that drawing. Find the measurement in the column at the left of the adjoining table, then note the corresponding number in the column having the color of the figure you chose. A 30-year-old woman—red figure—with a 29-inch abdomen would note the red number, 39.*

Step 1 table

inch	Women 35 and younger	Women 36 and older	Men 35 and younger	Men 36 and older
7"			26	
8"			30	
9"			33	
10"			37	
11"			41	
12"			44	
13"			48	
14"			52	
15"			56	
16"			59	
17"			63	
18"			67	
19"			70	
20"	27		74	
21"	28		78	
22"	29		81	
23"	31			
24"	32			
25"	33	30		
26"	35	31		
27"	36	32		
28"	37	33		29
29"	39	34		30
30"	40	36		31
31"	41	37		32
32"	43	38		34
33"	44	39		35
34"	45	40		36
35"	47	42		37
36"	48	43		38
37"	49	44		39
38"	51	45		40
39"	52	46		41
40"	53	48		42
41"		49		43
42"		50		44
43"		51		45
44"		52		46
45"		53		47
46"				48
47"				49
48"				50
49"				51

Step 2 table

inch	Women 35 and younger	Women 36 and older	Men 35 and younger	Men 36 and older
14"	29	17		
15"	31	19		
16"	33	20		
17"	35	21		
18"	37	22		
19"	40	23		
20"	42	25		
21"	44	26	28	
22"	46	27	29	
23"	48	28	30	
24"	50	30	31	
25"	52	31	33	
26"	54	32	34	23
27"	56	33	35	24
28"	58	35	37	25
29"	60	36	38	26
30"	62	37	39	27
31"	65	38	41	28
32"	67	40	42	29
33"	69	41	43	30
34"	71	42	45	30
35"			46	31
36"			47	32
37"			49	33
38"			50	34
39"			51	35
40"			52	36
41"			54	37
42"			55	38
43"				39
44"				39
45"				40
46"				41
47"				42

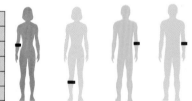

STEP 2: *Measure yourself again as indicated in the colored drawing (above) for your sex and age, and then find the corresponding number in the table at left. Add this number to the one that you noted in Step 1. If the woman in the example at Step 1 had a thigh measurement of 18 inches, she would add the number 37 to 39 (obtained in Step 1), for a sum of 76.*

Step 3 table

inch	Women 35 and younger	Women 36 and older	Men 35 and younger	Men 36 and older
6"	26			
7"	30		38	21
8"	34		43	24
9"	39		49	27
10"	43	14	54	30
11"	47	16	60	33
12"	52	17	65	36
13"	56	19	71	39
14"	60	20	76	42
15"	65	22	81	45
16"	69	23	87	48
17"	73	25	92	51
18"	78	26	98	54
19"	82	27	103	57
20"	86	29	109	60
21"	91	30	114	
22"		32	119	
23"		33		
24"		35		
25"		36		

STEP 3: *Take a third measurement (drawings above) and find the corresponding number in the table at left. Subtract this number from the sum derived in Steps 1 and 2. If the woman in the continuing example had an eight-inch forearm, she would subtract the number 34 from 76, leaving 42.*

STEP 4: *Finally, note the number printed in your color below—for a 30-year-old woman, number 20. Subtract it from the total of the first three steps. The result is the percentage of body fat for a sedentary person. If you exercise more than four hours a week, reduce this figure by 3 for a woman, by 4 for a man. If the woman in the example is sedentary, her body contains 22 per cent fat; if she exercises, 19 per cent.*

| 20 | 18 | 10 | 15 |

[ ] + [ ] − [ ] − [ ] = [ ] **% BODY FAT**

monly have much lower levels of testosterone than men.

Muscle size, in any case, is not the only index of strength. Physiologists have discovered several other ways in which muscles are strengthened by exercise. First, they become more efficient in handling the energy required for muscular effort. When muscles move they use energy released by a complex chain of chemical events in which the body converts food into the fuel that the muscles need for contraction. The body's capacity to change food into energy for the muscles improves drastically with regular exercise. In addition, the nerve-cell end plates (the part of the nerve that attaches to a muscle cell) become larger, making better electrical connections between nerve and muscle cells to transmit the impulses that cause muscles to contract on demand. Exercise also trains nerve and muscle cells to work in unison, like a seasoned drill team; thus there is less wasted effort.

Taking off flab

Besides making it possible for your body to withstand the rigors of life, exercises that produce stronger muscles can also help you bridge the gulf between the physique that you aspire to and the one that you confront every day in the mirror. They can help you bridge the gulf, but they cannot eliminate it. Body reshaping is accomplished in ways that are often misunderstood, and it is limited by factors that often go unrecognized. The basic shape of the human body is determined not by exercise or diet, but by the structure of bones and muscles, and by the distribution of fat.

Physiologists divide people into three basic body types. The endomorph generally has a broad trunk, relatively short limbs and a round face. The mesomorph has broad shoulders and a broad trunk with well-proportioned limbs, and he tends to be muscular. This is the physique considered the athletic shape. The ectomorph has a narrow trunk and long, thin limbs and face. Many distance runners are ectomorphs. Most people do not fall neatly into a single category, but rather are a combination of types. Yet each has a basic configuration given by bone and muscle structure, and little can be done to change it in any important way.

In fact, many of the claims about the effectiveness of body-shaping techniques are not true. No machine ever made, for example, will jiggle away an unwanted patch of fat, firm your muscles or change your basic contours while you relax and let it work. No set of exercises can selectively remove fat from precisely where you want it removed. You can certainly exercise enough to remove body fat. But the metabolic machinery at work inside your body will decide which cells will be called upon to give up their fat stores. And the cells tapped for their fat stores will not necessarily lie next to the muscles you are exercising.

This phenomenon was demonstrated in 1971 when researchers at the University of California at Orange measured the girths of the arms of a number of tennis players. In right-handed players the right arm, because of its heavy work load, was on the average one half inch greater in circumference than the left. Yet analysis of the layers of fat showed that they were identical on both arms. All the exercising had had no effect on the fat deposits in the exercised arm. Similarly, stomach exercises do not necessarily trim the stomach, nor do chin exercises always remove an extra chin.

However, stomach exercises can help eliminate a paunch and restore the middle of the body to its youthful form, and chin exercises can help remove unsightly neck sags. Other exercises will change the shape of other parts of the body. To some extent the changes can be targeted as desired. This is possible because different exercises affect different parts of the body in predictable ways—partly depending on sex.

Men, but generally not women, can reshape certain parts of their bodies by enlarging muscles. When men exercise specific muscles, those muscles increase in size. Competitive body builders demonstrate what this technique, carried to its limit, can do. Weight training, using barbells or elaborate health-club machines, is the exercise of choice here.

Great increases in muscle size are seldom the goal, even of men, in improving body shape. Most men and women aim to return to youthful proportions and posture. The slumps and sags that come with age can be straightened out by muscle-strengthening exercises, which create taut, firm tissue. Exercises that firm and strengthen the stomach muscles may flatten the stomach; in doing so they may also trim several inches from the waist measurement, even though they may not remove fat from that area. Strengthening the upper-shoulder, back and spinal muscles may correct a slumped, round-shouldered posture. For these purposes, calisthenics, which exercise all the principal muscle groups, are just as effective as weight training.

Yet firm muscles are only part of a shapely physique. Weight, and particularly the distribution of weight, is the overwhelming influence on the form of the body. When most people look in a mirror, they see too much of themselves. It is common for Americans who were trim in their youth to gain weight at the rate of one half to one pound per year after their 20th birthday. Most of the added bulk is fat, and much of the surplus fat develops where it detracts from appearance. In men, fat accumulates mostly around the middle, in the abdomen and buttocks. Women build up fat there, and also in the arms and thighs. These are the parts of the body that most people would prefer to have slimmer. Thus the best way to improve body shape generally is to get rid of excess fat.

Not everyone who looks heavy, however, is too fat—the structure and size of bones and muscles are major factors. To determine if eliminating fat will produce significant changes in your own appearance, you must determine how much fat your body contains and compare this with ideal amounts. A man in good condition should have about 15 per cent of his total weight in fat. A woman needs no more than about 25 per cent body fat. Most people tend to put on fat with age. This is not good for health, and the figures given here are goals recommended regardless of age.

Unfortunately, the traditional methods for helping you judge your fat content are not reliable. In fact, your mirror, your scale and the common weight charts can all be mislead-

Why golf will not help you lose weight

Exercise can help you shed excess weight if it makes you expend more energy in physical activity than you get from the food you eat. Some exercises are better than others as reducing aids, and some help hardly at all. This graph compares the rate at which calories (food energy) are consumed by 11 popular activities.

Best for reducing are endurance exercises such as running and bicycling, which burn calories faster than the others. In the middle of the scale is singles tennis—assuming the players have the skill to keep the ball in play and energy to get going again quickly when one of them misses. Least effective is golf. Even if a golfer walks the course and carries his clubs, the game consumes only 300 calories per hour. (A golfer who rides a golf cart uses only half as many calories, about the same amount required for an hour of typing.) The graph applies to a person weighing 150 pounds; the calorie-consumption figures increase or decrease 10 per cent for every 15 pounds' difference in weight.

Activity	Calories
Bicycling (15 miles per hour)	~730
Running (6 miles per hour)	~660
Swimming (40 yards per minute)	~550
Basketball	~560
Soccer	~555
Football	~550
Tennis (singles)	~450
Volleyball	~350
Walking (4 miles per hour)	~330
Tennis (doubles)	~320
Golf (walking and carrying clubs)	~300

CALORIES CONSUMED PER HOUR
0 100 200 300 400 500 600 700 800

ing. According to the charts, a burly professional football player might be as much as 75 to 80 pounds overweight. In all likelihood, however, he would be leaner than most other people. What is important is not a comparison of weight, height and age—the standards applied in most charts—but an accurate appraisal of how much fat your body contains.

A precise measurement of body fat requires laboratory equipment. You sit on a seat—like a child's swing—suspended from a scale, and a laboratory technician records your weight. Then, after exhaling to empty your lungs, you are lowered into a tank of water and completely submerged for a few seconds so that the technician can measure your weight underwater. These two weight measurements are used to calculate both the volume of your body and its density—that is, how much it weighs per cubic centimeter or cubic inch. This information, when compared with the known density of fat and the density of the body's other tissues, tells just how many pounds of fat your body contains.

Although such hydrostatic weighing is the most reliable method of determining body fat, you can make a reasonably accurate estimate at home with a simple series of measurements and calculations, shown on pages 44-45.

If your own percentage of fat turns out to be higher than the ideal percentage for your sex, exercise, preferably in combination with a reducing diet, can probably alter the shape of your body for the better—slimming the middle and, in women, the arms and thighs. Exercise and diet eliminate fat by reversing the process that caused it to accumulate. Food provides nutrients that are converted into energy for powering active muscles. If you do not burn up what you eat, the excess becomes fat. Conversely, if you burn up more than you eat, the fat deposits are reduced. If the deficit between food intake and the consumption of food by exercise is just 500 calories per day, you will remove about a pound of fat a week.

Either diet or exercise alone will get rid of fat, but the two work better and faster together. Even a good diet is much more pleasant and rewarding if you supplement it with exercise, which not only forces your body to burn more fat but makes your muscles firmer so that they will not hang slack from your frame as you become thinner.

Indeed, once you start exercising you may be tempted to get rid of all extra fat with exercise. But you can see from the chart on page 47 how hard you would have to exercise to burn up just 500 calories a day. Even if you are capable of exercising at such a strenuous pace when you first begin—and most people are not—you would lose a pound a week only if your weight was stable before you ran, pedaled or swam the first mile. If you are gaining weight without exercise, it is impractical to shed pounds quickly with exercise alone.

Any exercise—whether walking, calisthenics or weight training—burns calories. And any diet will help, so long as it is sensibly balanced and limited in quantity. (Crash diets are counterproductive, often retarding fat loss: The body, reacting to apparent starvation, tries to conserve its store of nutrients by slowing the rate at which it converts them to energy.)

A man who combines exercise with diet may not immediately take weight off. He may gain a few pounds at first. The explanation for this seeming lack of progress is a simple one. Exercise builds larger muscles at the same time that, and often at a faster rate than, it burns fat. Thus when a man begins exercising, the bathroom scales show the same or more weight instead of less and they may continue to do so for several weeks, until exercise has enlarged the muscles about as much as it is going to. At that point weight will stabilize and begin to go down. But even while weight refuses to decrease, measurements shrink, reshaping the body, because muscle is more compact than the fat it replaces.

Some women encounter a similar effect: Their bodies become more compact even though they may not lose a single pound. Joan Ullyot, a San Francisco physician and marathon runner, had just that experience in her early thirties, after she started exercising. "In five years of running," she said, "even though I haven't lost any weight, my pants size has gone from 14 to 10."

Supple muscles, limber joints

The misconception is all too common that a sleek body, strength and stamina are all that are needed for fitness. Ballet dancers, who have all these attributes, have always known better. Many of the warm-up exercises that they have per-

Measuring flexibility with a stretch test

You can gauge your flexibility approximately but simply with a test devised by the YMCA: While seated on the floor bend forward from the waist and see how far you can stretch—without discomfort—noting the distance on a measuring stick *(right, bottom)*. The average Y member, among the 2,100 who took part in development of the test, could reach about a foot or a foot and a half if he was a middle-aged man, somewhat farther if a woman.

This stretch test is used to help identify YMCA applicants whose inability to bend freely at the waist may indicate tightness in the hamstrings and in the muscles of the lower back—a common cause of backache. Applicants who rate no better than "fair" according to the norms in the table below are offered stretching exercises similar to the ones illustrated on pages 95-96, which limber those crucial muscles.

The Y's test is admittedly crude. It gauges only one joint—the hip—giving an incomplete measure of body flexibility. And the standards against which you gauge your own performance can be misleading, for they are based on the abilities of YMCA members, who may be in better condition than the general population. Still, the test provides a quick and easy way to indicate how much stretching exercises may help you.

HOW TO TAKE THE FLEXIBILITY TEST
Draw or tape a line on the floor and place a measuring stick across it so that the line is even with the 15-inch mark. Sit on the floor so that your heels are on the line and your feet are about five inches apart (above). With your legs straight, bend forward as far as you comfortably can, and touch the stick (right). Caution: Do not jerk forward; you could strain your back or leg muscles. The mark you reach is your score; the chart below rates performance for men and women of three age groups.

Rating Flexibility by Inches of Stretch

	Age 35 and younger		Age 36-45		Age 46 and older	
	MEN	WOMEN	MEN	WOMEN	MEN	WOMEN
Excellent	21″ or more	23″ or more	20″ or more	22″ or more	19″ or more	21″ or more
Good	15″-20″	18″-22″	14″-19″	17″-21″	13″-18″	16″-20″
Fair	8″-14″	12″-17″	6″-13″	11″-16″	6″-12″	10″-15″
Poor	7″ or less	11″ or less	5″ or less	10″ or less	5″ or less	9″ or less

formed at the bar for centuries are intended to provide another quality. The dancers stretch their muscles to keep them long and pliable, enabling the joints to move freely and easily. These exercises are among the simplest to perform. They require only extension of the limbs and bending and swinging of movable parts of the body *(Chapter 3),* limbering its connections to improve its flexibility.

In recent years, professional athletes have come to recognize the value of such stretching exercises. Each football season the Pittsburgh Steelers were plagued with muscle pulls and strains. Suspecting that the injury rate might be lowered by a conditioning program that was more refined than the calisthenics, running and weight training the athletes were accustomed to, the team hired Paul Uram, a high-school football coach, in 1973. Uram came to the Steelers' attention because of research he had done to determine the effects of various kinds of exercises on the performance of athletes in a number of sports, and he devised for the Steelers a program of stretching exercises, unusual for football players at that time, to supplement their regular workouts.

During the next few seasons, the number of pulled muscles and similar self-inflicted injuries began to decline, a trend that Uram feels contributed to the four Super Bowl victories that the Steelers chalked up during the next seven years.

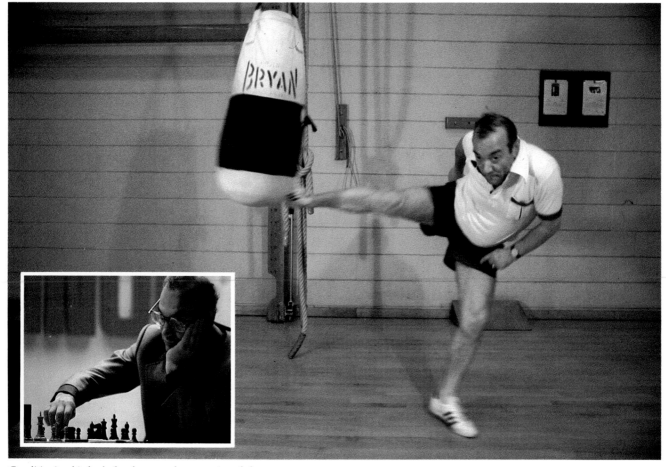

Conditioning his body for the mental gymnastics of chess, Russian master Viktor Korchnoi delivers a high kick to a punching bag. World-class chess is so fatiguing that contenders of Korchnoi's age (here in his late 40s) are rare. To relax their muscles and increase their stamina, most chess champions follow regular programs of physical exercise.

Other teams have had similar success in reducing injuries by including stretching exercises in their pregame warm-up.

These exercises protect against injury because they increase the capacity of joints to move. Some joints, like the one in the shoulder, move in many directions with nearly equal facility. Others, like those in the knees and elbows, flex in one direction only. Still other joints, the ones in the spine for example, have a very limited range of motion. But like strength and stamina, the joints' various ranges of motion diminish with inactivity.

This loss of limberness begins at an early age. "Once kids start riding the school bus," said Bob Spackman, Professor of Physical Education at Southern Illinois University, "they forget they have legs. I can pick 100 boys eight to 12 years old and probably not one of them will be able to put his palms on the floor with his knees locked." This inflexibility grows worse with age as physical activity steadily decreases; the more sedentary a person's life, the greater the stiffness.

Loss of flexibility can be counteracted by stretching, according to Herbert deVries, Professor of Physical Education at the University of Southern California, because it works on the sheath of connective tissue, called the fascia, that encases a muscle. When a muscle fascia is immobilized by disuse or injury, it becomes shorter and less pliant, restricting the length of the muscle and limiting the movements of the joint that the muscle controls. Gently stretching a muscle can lengthen the fascia and enhance freedom of movement.

Furthermore, said deVries, a shortened fascia places "undue pressure on nerve pathways located in the fascia. The result is that many aches and pains are the result of nerve impulses traveling along the already pressured pathways." Whether muscle aches are caused by a taut fascia or by a pressured nerve pathway, they can be soothed by stretching. Nighttime cramps in the calves, for example, often can be eliminated simply by stretching.

Even muscles that have been hurt in sports competition can be helped by stretching. DeVries invited injured athletes to his laboratory, where he measured the electrical signals sent out by their sore muscles. A fully extended and relaxed muscle emits no impulses, but the injured muscles of the athletes showed a high level of electrical activity, indicating shortening and tension. The athletes were next taught to stretch their aching muscles. Afterward the electrical impulses in the same muscles were counted again and found to be fewer in number, an indication that stretching had reduced muscle tension. At the same time, the athletes reported that their pains had subsided.

Balm for frazzled nerves

Tight muscles arise from many causes besides injury—foremost among them fatigue and emotional tension—and stretching is only one of many exercises that relax the tightness. In another experiment, deVries found that a "moderate, 15-minute walk" resulted in greater relaxation in his subjects' muscles than did a normal dose of tranquilizer, and the exercise produced none of the drug's side effects.

Many people who exercise after a hard day at work feel that the relaxation of their muscles promotes an overall sensation of tranquillity. They say they come back from a run or a swim feeling calmed. A few sets of tennis, a handball match, a round of golf, or a game of volleyball may have the same effect: Tense muscles relax, and the cares and worries of the day seem to disperse like smoke in a breeze.

Of all the methods of achieving relaxation through exercise, however, the most famous is the one intended specifically for this purpose: the traditional hatha-yoga of the Orient. These combinations of bodily position and spiritual concentration turn the practitioner's attention inward, far from the stresses and strains of daily endeavors.

Yet the purpose of yoga is not solely relaxation. Its proponents claim that it has many other values as well. One manual, typical of treatises on the subject, says that yoga's "physical training brings strength, grace and suppleness; tones up circulation, internal organs; regulates weight; influences height; increases vital energy." That list of yogic consequences sounds remarkably like the claims made by Western experts in the field of exercise. Physical fitness, although it can be divided into distinct components, is really just one thing—a condition of well-being that makes life more worth living. ✸

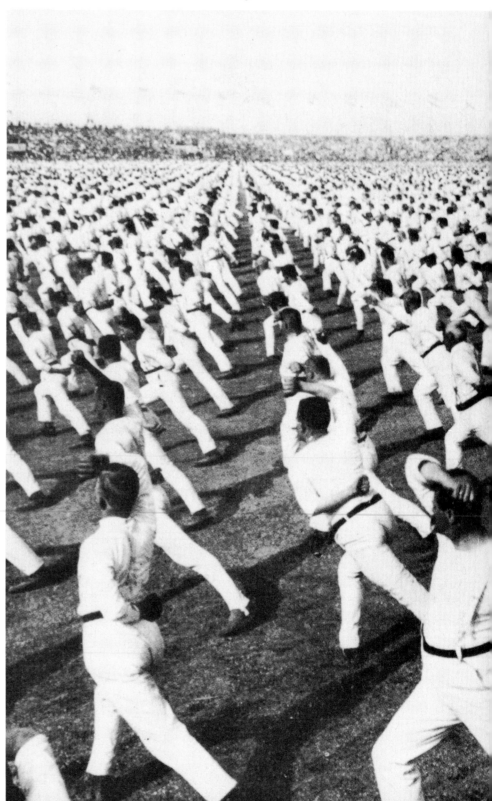

Reviving the Greek ideal of mind and body

"A sound mind in a manly body." So said the Greek poet Homer, when asked to name a man's greatest blessing. He was expressing the classical view of men as whole beings whose intellectual, physical and spiritual development should harmonize. Yet, with the death of classical society, training of the mind and of the spirit was emphasized and physical exercise was neglected. Not until the Age of Enlightenment did philosophers re-adopt the view that a man was incomplete if his body went untrained.

One of the first to recognize the implications of this philosophical change was a fierce Prussian patriot by the name of Friedrich Ludwig Jahn, a Berlin schoolteacher who is considered a father of modern exercise programs. In 1807 Jahn, dismayed when Napoleon destroyed the independence of Prussia, set out to rekindle national pride. He led bands of his young pupils into the countryside for group exercises and lectures. His aim was partly physical improvement and partly the inspiration of patriotism and resistance to foreign imperialism.

Jahn's methods and message drew hundreds to his cause. In 1814, a year after Napoleon's defeat in Germany, Jahn organized a gymnastics festival, or *turnfest*. In time, the *turnfests* would become national events.

Jahn was not the only one to recognize the value of mass exercise. Eighteenth and 19th Century feminists, religious leaders, educators, factory managers and military leaders began to employ group exercises to serve their various purposes. And, ironically, in Jahn's native land, nearly a century after the first anti-imperialist *turnfest*, the Kaiser's warlike regime used exercise to rally people in support of its imperialistic goals *(right)*.

Some 17,000 men exercise together at the 12th German Gymnastics Festival in Leipzig a year before the outbreak of World War I. The Kaiser's regime staged the festival to display German power and unity.

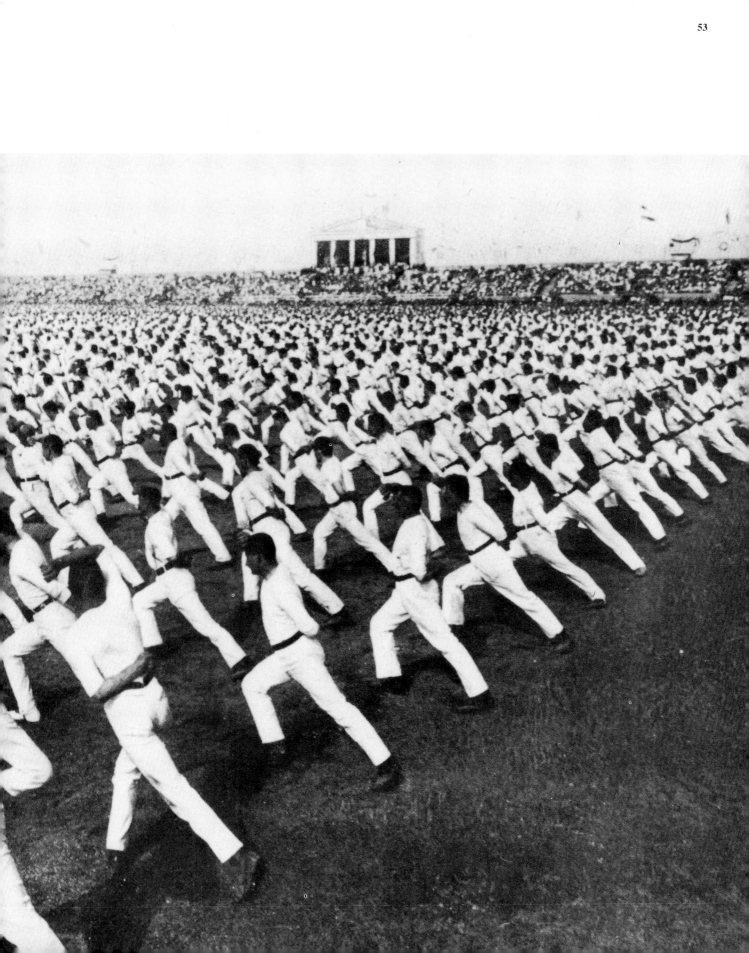

Overcoming the myth of feminine frailty

The Victorian ideal of womanhood held that exercise was unladylike; many doctors believed it was positively damaging to the feminine constitution. Wrote Dr. Edward Hammond Clarke of Boston: "Woman, in the interest of the race, is dowered with a set of organs peculiar to herself. If neglected and mismanaged, they retaliate upon their possessor with weakness and disease."

To Catharine E. Beecher, headmistress of a Connecticut girls' school, such contentions were preposterous. In 1831 she introduced exercises called calisthenics, from the Greek for "beautiful," *kalos,* and for "strength," *sthenos.* Beecher later toured the country, convincing thousands that exercise was vital for women. By 1900, most schools offered fitness courses to female students, and such women's colleges as Mount Holyoke, Smith and Vassar taught calisthenics.

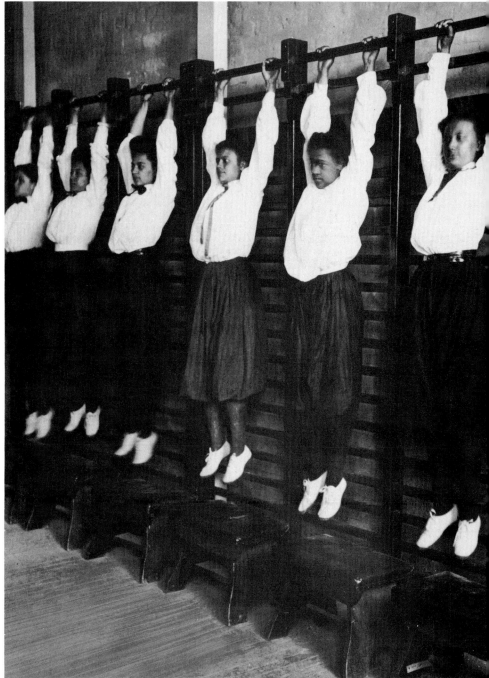

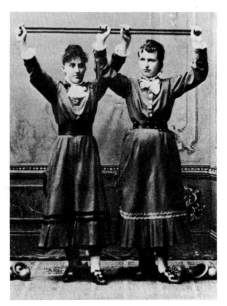

Two women at Smith College in 1879 use a long wand to help them exercise. Holding the wand overhead, the women bent in unison from side to side to stretch and strengthen the muscles of their trunks.

Six students at the Negro Women's Seminary dangle from gymnastic ladders in 1906. This stretching routine was intended to improve posture; on command, the students raised their legs forward to tone and strengthen their stomach muscles.

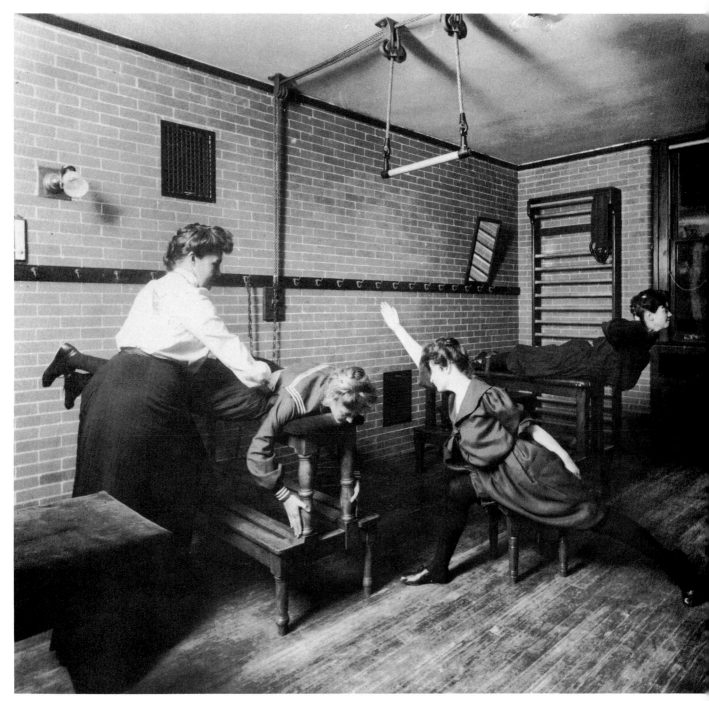

A physical education instructor in the gymnasium of Teacher's
College in New York shows a 1904 student how to do an exercise
that uses a bench. At rear, a second pupil works on flexibility
while a third exercises to strengthen her lower back.

The YMCA: linking moral and physical fitness

In its work of steering young men, fresh off the farm, away from the pool halls and saloons of 19th Century cities, the Young Men's Christian Association in 1856 added exercise to the religious and intellectual programs it had provided since its inception in London 12 years earlier. "Any machinery," stated the Y, "will be incomplete which has not taken into account the whole man."

In 1869 the first two YMCA gymnasiums opened, in New York and San Francisco. By 1887 there were nearly 170 in the United States, by 1900 more than 500, involving 80,000 young men in organized exercise.

There was good reason for the strong turnout: Many of the Y gyms were among the best in the world. New York's 23rd Street Y, for example, cost the then-princely sum of a half million dollars to build in 1869. Almost all of the gyms had such standard gear as punching bags, parallel bars, horizontal bars, rowing machines and dumbbells. Many employed trained physical directors—some of whom were former circus acrobats and professional athletes. Toward the turn of the century, the best of the YMCA facilities had indoor swimming pools and the newest had courts for two games recently invented by Y officials: volleyball and basketball.

Exercise enthusiasts of the late 19th Century pause during their workouts at a YMCA gymnasium. Though cramped, this gym offered patrons a variety of equipment: parallel bars, flying rings, a Roman ladder for making a human pyramid (rear), horizontal bars, a punching bag and hydraulic rowing machines (foreground). Lighter exercises were done with the rings, bars, wands, barbells, and Indian clubs hanging on the wall at right.

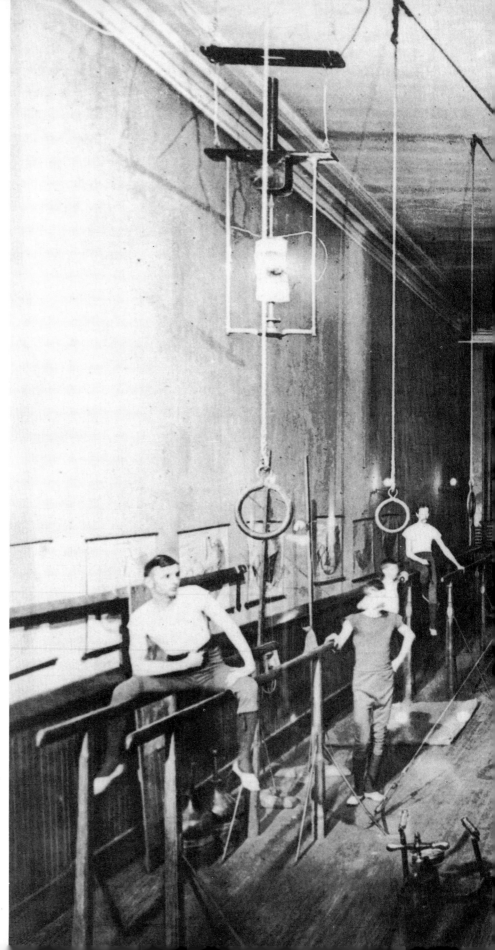

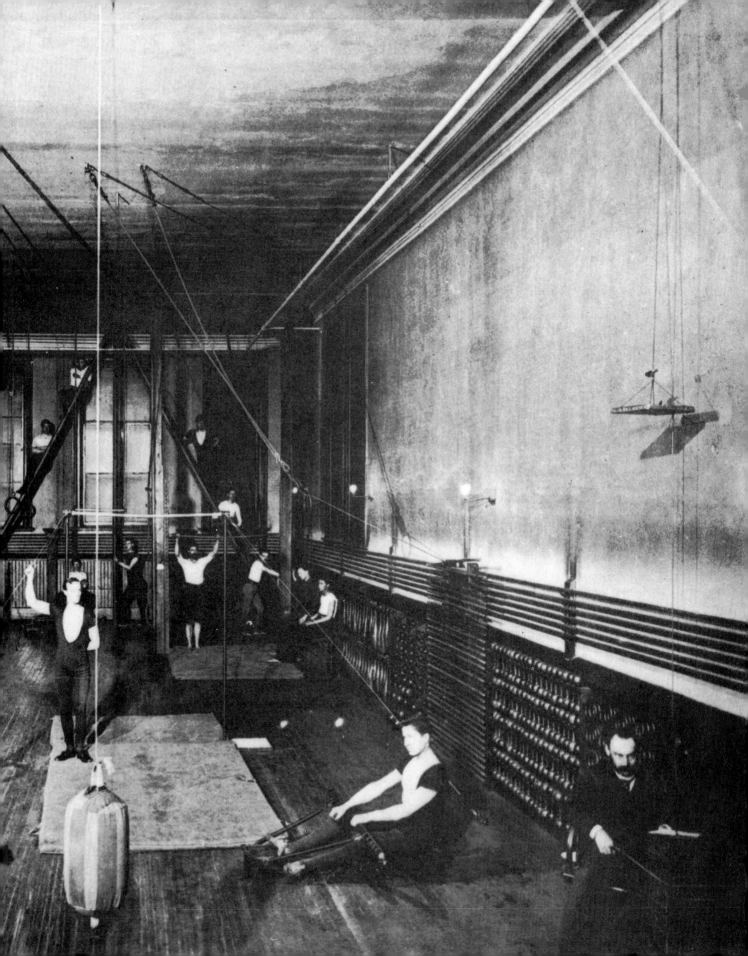

In the classroom, education for the body

"The great secret of education," wrote the French philosopher Jean Jacques Rousseau in 1762, "is to make the exercises of the body and of the mind always serve as recreation for each other." Rousseau's call for combining intellectual and physical education went unheeded in his own land, but not in Germany. In Dessau in 1774, a generation before Friedrich Ludwig Jahn made exercise a mass activity *(pages 52-53)*, the progressive academy called the Philanthropinum instituted the first school courses in physical education.

Students of the Philanthropinum spent an hour in the morning and two in the afternoon in sports and gymnastics. At first, they were encouraged by their teachers to run, jump, fence and wrestle. Soon instructors began to teach swimming and skating.

The example of the Philanthropinum was slow to be followed in other schools. Conservative educators thought that schooltime was no time for such "play," and many considered physical activity somehow sinful. Others felt that youngsters got plenty of healthful exercise from manual labor.

Nevertheless, schools in the United States and Europe gradually added exercise to the curriculum. In 1827, the Round Hill School in Northampton, Massachusetts, hired America's first physical education teacher—a German political refugee familiar with the methods pioneered at the Philanthropinum. In the 1850s, the public schools of Boston became the first in the United States to require daily exercise, and in 1867 Philadelphia directed teachers "to devote in each school room ten minutes during the course of each school session to such physical exercises as the size of the room . . . might permit." Usually that meant desk-side calisthenics like those being practiced at right.

By the start of the 20th Century, most big-city schools in the United States had rules requiring at least 50 minutes of exercise a week. In Chicago in 1900, seven of the 15 high schools had fully-equipped gyms.

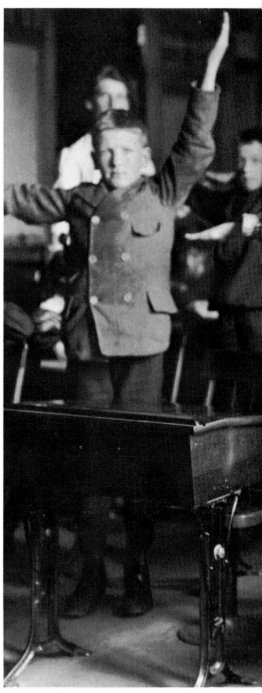

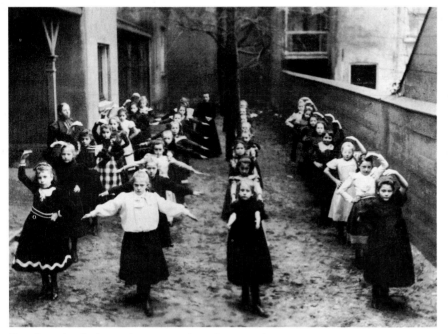

Fourth graders in Amsterdam are put through an exercise routine by two stern teachers (left and rear) around 1910. In many schools in Europe and the United States, such calisthenics were, even in the 20th Century, one of the few types of exercise deemed appropriate for schoolgirls; more vigorous activities remained largely the exclusive province of boys.

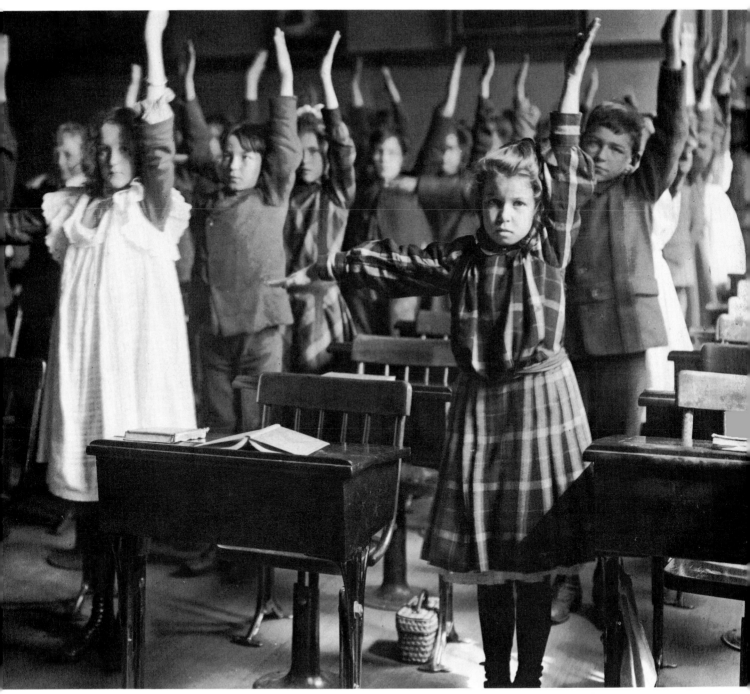

School children perform calisthenics at their desks in Brockton, Massachusetts, in the early 1900s. Sitting for many hours at school desks, wrote one exercise advocate of the day, "is biologically abnormal" and should "be met by frequent breaks throughout the day." At such times, he wrote, students could "vigorously exercise the muscles which counteract desk attitude."

Calisthenics on the job: "It pays"

John H. Patterson, the founder of the National Cash Register company, gave an admirably straight answer when anyone asked him why he had his employees exercise on company time: "It pays," he said.

Patterson had not always felt that way. Until 1894, recalled *Forbes* magazine years later, Patterson had been "neither better nor worse than other factory owners. His interest in his employees was confined to what he could get out of them."

However, the magazine continued, Patterson had a change of heart. He provided his employees with lockers, fresh coffee, and clean water for washing. And he scheduled exercise periods *(right)*—twice daily, for 10 minutes, at 10 a.m. and 3 p.m. As soon as the exercise program was instituted, noted a contemporary company newsletter, management and employees alike discovered that fewer people reported sick and that "the power for work increased."

Patterson was not the first modern businessman to see the implications of physical fitness for industry. Heads of other companies in the United States and Europe—particularly in Germany—had arrived at similar conclusions. In 1884, Krupp, Germany's largest steelmaker, organized a gymnastics and fencing club. Later, Luftschiffbau Zeppelin, the airship builders, opened a company gymnasium and the giant Bayer chemical company set up an exercise hall for use by its employees *(below)*.

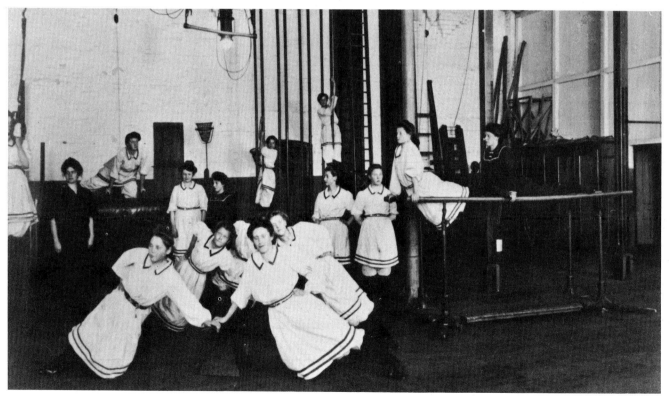

Female workers at Germany's Friedrich Bayer & Co. work out in 1904 in a storage room converted to a gymnasium. Bayer also sponsored other activities, including soccer and boxing for men, but the little gym was a special point of corporate pride: When the Deputy Emperor of China visited the company in 1908, the highlight of his tour was a visit to the gym.

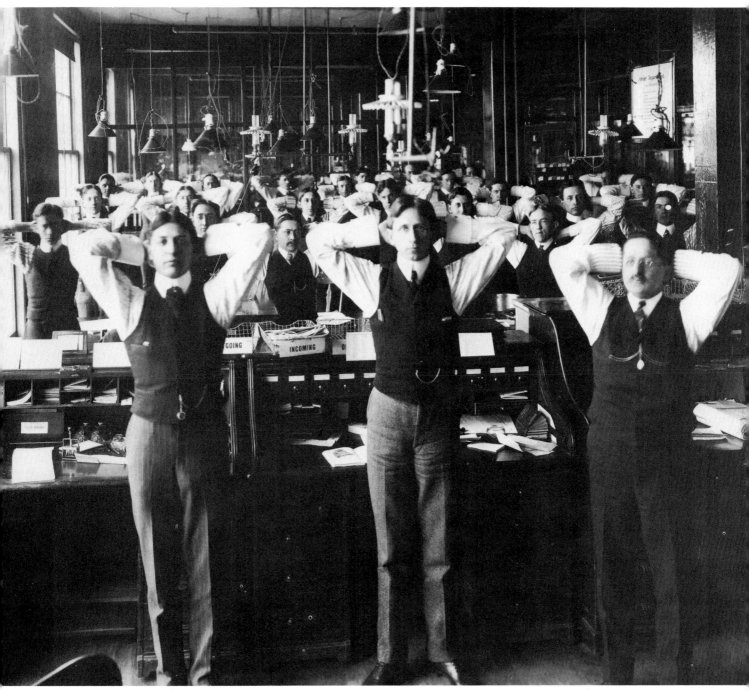

Men in the order department of the National Cash Register company perform their morning calisthenics in February 1902. The company also opened a gymnasium for employees to use after business hours. Its equipment included a rowing machine and a newfangled electric contrivance that, boasted a company newsletter, simulated "all the exercise of camel riding."

Ensuring that soldier and sailor are able to fight

As late as 1917, the United States armed services paid scant attention to physical fitness. The military had no officially sanctioned exercise program. There were occasional ball games and athletic competitions, and particularly conscientious officers might order their men to do calisthenics *(right),* but the basic military assumption was that the men were fit enough without formal exercise. World War I changed that thinking.

At induction, the Army found that 35 per cent of its recruits were physically unfit. In training camp, nearly 30 per cent of the soldiers of one regiment were unable to jump across trenches six feet wide; in another unit, 17 per cent were unable to sprint 220 yards in less than 30 seconds.

To improve the men's fitness, military leaders instituted physical training programs at bases in the United States and abroad. Soldiers and sailors entered a two-track conditioning regimen: Half of the training consisted of marching, drill and calisthenics; the other half emphasized sports and games, such as boxing and wrestling, baseball and football, and track-and-field events.

By the end of World War I, the Army and Navy had become, in terms of numbers and intensity of commitment, the world's staunchest boosters of physical fitness. "We have had a clinical opportunity to study the matter of physical training," said United States Secretary of War Newton D. Baker in 1919, and "it goes without saying that the strength of a nation in the last analysis depends upon the physical vigor, the mental vigor, and the morale of its young men."

Sailors aboard the armored cruiser U.S.S. New York touch their toes in 1899 while their goat mascot watches. Such organized exercises were comparatively rare in the turn-of-the-century Navy; most officers gave little thought to the amount of shipboard exercise their subordinates got.

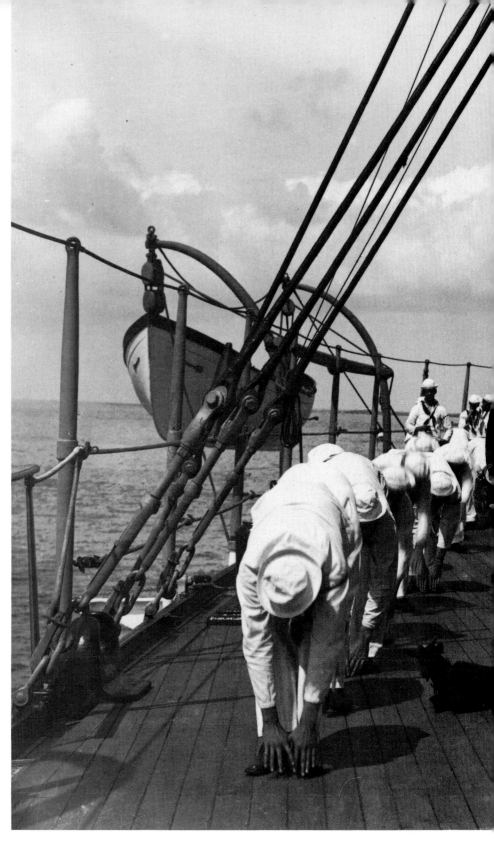

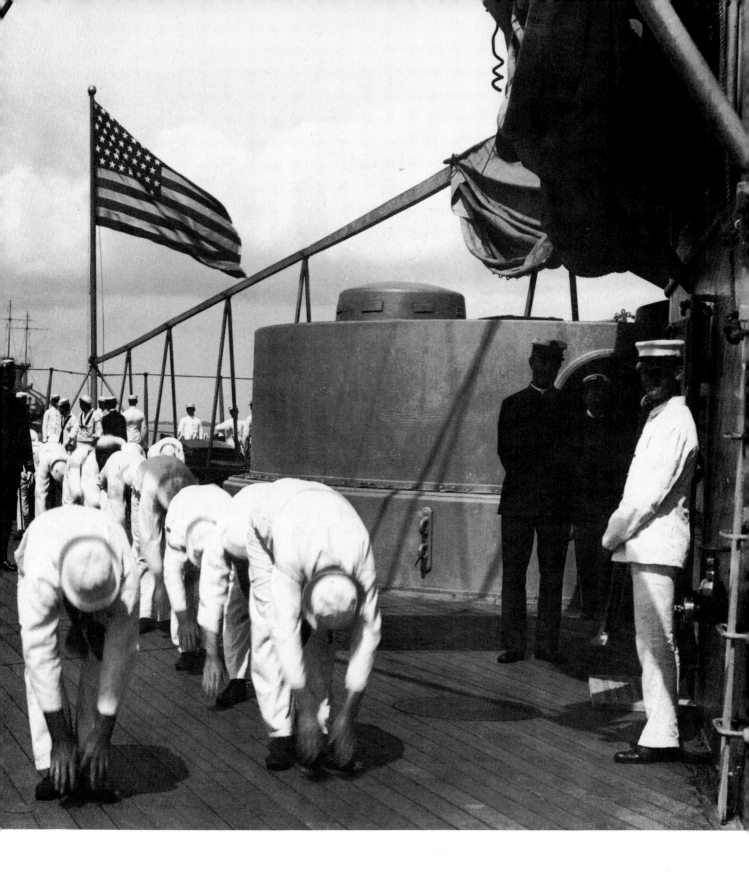

CHAPTER 3

Techniques for keeping fit

A question of safety
Who needs a stress test
Choosing an endurance exercise
Toward a trimmer physique
Building strong muscles
Easing tensions away

On a flight from New Orleans to New York, the pilot heard a steady thumping sound. He checked all the instruments but was unable to find anything suspicious. He was sufficiently alarmed to consider turning around and going back to New Orleans, but at last the thumping stopped. After he had landed uneventfully in New York, one of the flight attendants stuck her head into the cockpit. "What a weird passenger we had on this flight," she said. "He locked himself in the forward lavatory and jogged in place for 20 minutes."

Not many people go to such lengths to find the time and a place for exercise. For most, regular exercise fits much more easily into the daily routine.

When you set out to exercise, you will face considerations more complex than time and place. They settle themselves once you know something about exercises and their effects on your health. Although there is a bewildering variety of exercises, choosing among them is simplified because all fall into only a few basic categories. The techniques of performing the exercises are not difficult to learn *(pages 92-112)*— you do not have to be a superbly coordinated athlete or dancer to profit from exercises. For most activities, you need little or no special equipment; even the mystique of the jogging shoe—there are 150 or more models—reduces to two or three practical considerations. Special diets and vitamin supplements are unnecessary; what is necessary is a good normal diet—whether you exercise or not.

You also need an understanding of the way you go about exercising: preparing your body to accommodate the stresses

that will be placed on it, pacing yourself to get the most from your efforts, and guarding against errors that can cause discomfort or injury.

Before you undertake regular exercises, you should reassure yourself that you can perform them safely. They will subject your body to more physical stress than it has been accustomed to—that is the whole point of exercising. Extra, unaccustomed stress can sometimes be dangerous, and you may need a medical checkup before you begin. Articles and books on exercise commonly recommend such an examination for everyone more than 35 years old. Many physicians, on the other hand, believe this recommendation is overcautious and impractical.

If you are in good health, there are many exercises you probably can begin safely without seeing a doctor. The decision in each case depends on the exercise and your age, weight and level of physical activity. The more vigorous the exercise, the more important a physical checkup becomes.

For example, if you are interested primarily in limbering your body or relaxing it, you can probably begin such routines at any time. These exercises must be performed slowly to succeed, so there is not much risk of injury to joints or muscles or of damage to your heart. Even the more strenuous varieties of exercise necessary for strengthening the heart and other muscles or for ridding the body of fat are also relatively safe for most people.

Yet you may be among the minority of apparently healthy men and women who should seek the advice of a physician

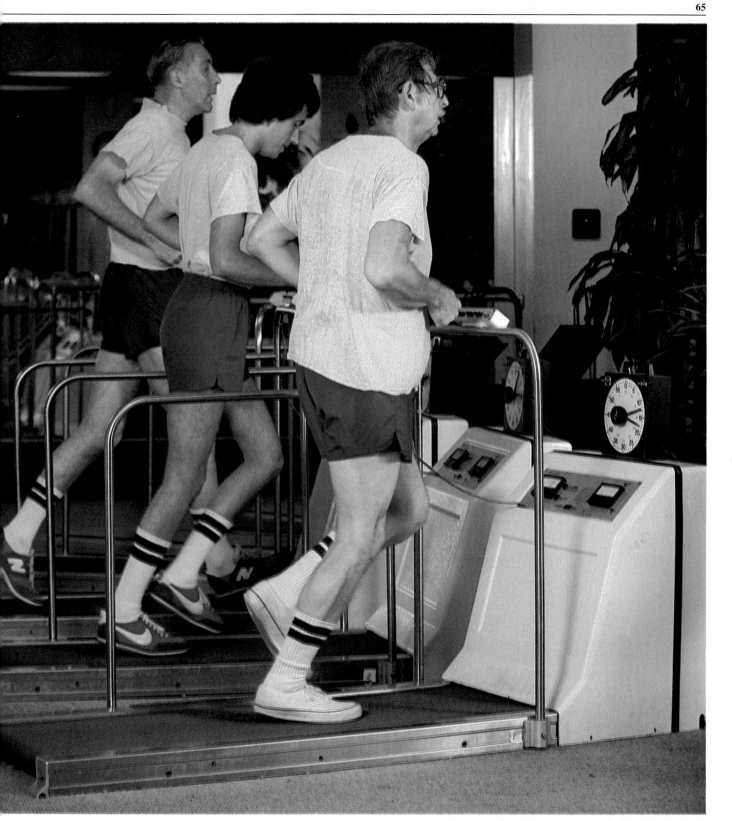

Joggers work on the automatic treadmills of Manhattan's Cardio-Fitness Center, one of the health clubs that have become an increasingly popular setting for exercise in the United States (pages 85-88). The speed and incline of the machines can be adjusted for runners of different levels of fitness; a timer and an odometer tell the duration and "distance" of a run.

before exercising toward any goal except flexibility or relaxation. There are several warning signs: back pain, discomfort in major joints such as the knees or shoulders, chest pains, shortness of breath, heart palpitations, dizziness or chronic headaches. If you are troubled by any of these symptoms and you have not already checked with your doctor about the problem, then you should do so before you attempt any program of vigorous exercise. The same advice applies if any of these symptoms are evident when you test your own physical fitness or at any time after you have begun exercising regularly.

Moreover, a consultation with your doctor is essential if you have ever been treated for a heart ailment—even if it has apparently been cured—or if you have a history of diabetes, high blood pressure or high levels of blood cholesterol. Though you should see your doctor, only in the rarest cases will any of these ailments prevent you from exercising. Indeed, over the long run exercise often lowers blood pressure and alleviates symptoms of heart disease.

An examination under stress

In most cases a doctor will be able to determine on the basis of an examination in his office how strenuously you can exercise. Sometimes, however, he may prescribe a more revealing stress test.

A doctor may put you through such a test in his office by having you climb and descend a special set of steps, but he is more likely to refer you to a stress-testing facility, usually in a hospital. There a blood pressure cuff—the pneumatic band the doctor inflates around your arm when he takes your blood pressure—is put in place, and an array of electrodes is attached to your chest to record heart signals in an electrocardiogram. Then you begin to exercise at a prescribed pace, on a treadmill or a stationary bicycle that can be adjusted to require increasing effort.

Gradually the work load is intensified. For example, you begin walking the treadmill at a leisurely pace, and eventually, as its speed is increased, you end up running. To raise your energy output even more, one end of the treadmill is elevated progressively to higher positions, so you are in ef-

fect running up a hill that gets steeper and steeper. As the test proceeds, the test physician monitors heart signals and checks blood pressure. Such a test simulates the rigors of vigorous exercises and can reveal circulatory disorders that are not always apparent in a doctor's office.

Who needs a stress test

A stress test may sound like a good idea for anyone ready to begin exercising, if only to be on the safe side. But the test is expensive and of little medical advantage for most people. Indeed, many doctors who are also avid exercisers do not attach much importance to the procedure. Three physicians from the Scott and White Clinic of Temple, Texas, all marathon runners themselves, sent questionnaires to the other physicians who had run with them in the 1978 Boston Marathon, asking each what he thought and what he did about pre-exercise stress testing and physical examination.

As the three reported in *The New England Journal of Medicine,* 83 per cent of the 69 responding doctors did not have stress tests before they began running, 66 per cent said they did not believe in giving stress tests to patients who displayed no symptoms of heart disease, and 45 per cent reported that they believed physical examination had been oversold to the public.

One reason that many doctors are unenthusiastic about stress tests is that they are unreliable. They often give false positives, indicating defects that further examinations prove nonexistent, or worse, they produce false negatives, failing to detect the presence of serious disabilities.

False positives are discouragingly common. When stress tests are administered to apparently healthy people, they often indicate heart disease; yet when those cases are subjected to more discriminating tests, 60 per cent of them are found to have sound hearts. Not only do such errors cause unnecessary concern, but they often lead to additional laboratory examinations that are expensive and superfluous.

Much more alarming are the false negatives. Some people who take stress tests are given a clean bill of health even though the coronary arteries, which supply blood to the heart, may be dangerously narrowed by deposits of choles-

A trail specially equipped for an outdoor workout

The path of fitness chosen by increasing numbers of Americans and Europeans is the exercise trail—a kind of open-air gymnasium that offers a variety of exercises to strengthen and limber muscles as well as improve the circulatory system. Invented in Switzerland, the trails were introduced to the United States in 1973 by a San Francisco firm, Parcourse, Ltd., but have since been adapted by others.

Fitness trails consist of 18 or so exercise stations. Beginning with easy warm-up exercises, the trails continue with progressively more strenuous strength-building exercises, followed by a stretching routine. Signs explain how to do each exercise and suggest how many times a beginning, intermediate or advanced exerciser should be able to repeat it. Between stations the heart gets a workout as exercisers walk, jog or bicycle.

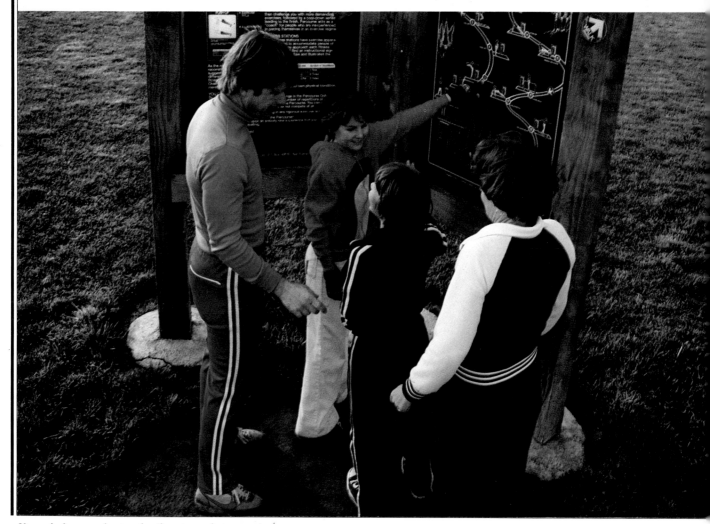

Up early for a workout, a family gets ready to exercise on a fitness trail in San Francisco. The signs behind them introduce the trail with a map and instructions. Signs also tell participants what to do—in this case, to walk to station No. 1.

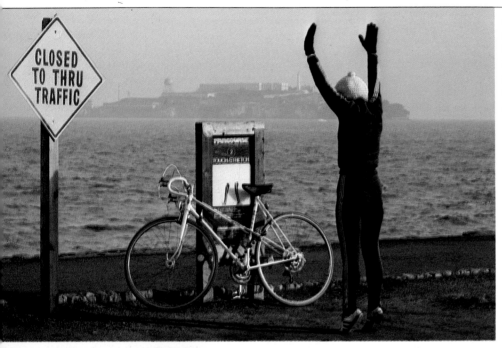

A bicyclist limbers up with a stretching exercise for leg, arm and trunk muscles at a trail station on San Francisco Bay, overlooking Alcatraz. Because stations are only 100 to 250 yards apart, bicycling between them does not provide as much exercise as walking or running.

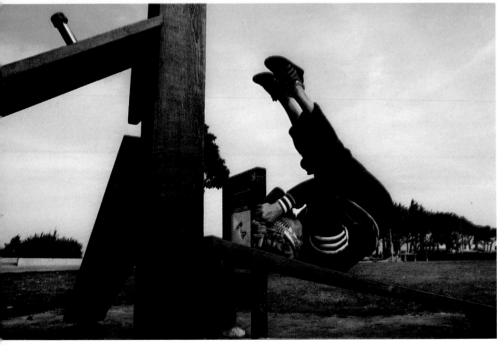

A slanted board with a handgrip made of steel pipe forms the simple apparatus for the body curl, an exercise that strengthens abdominal muscles. Two similar but steeper boards (center and left) pose a bigger challenge as exercisers toughen muscles.

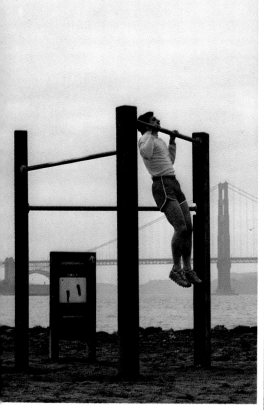

At a station halfway through the San Francisco course—with the Golden Gate Bridge in the background—are chinning bars positioned at various heights.

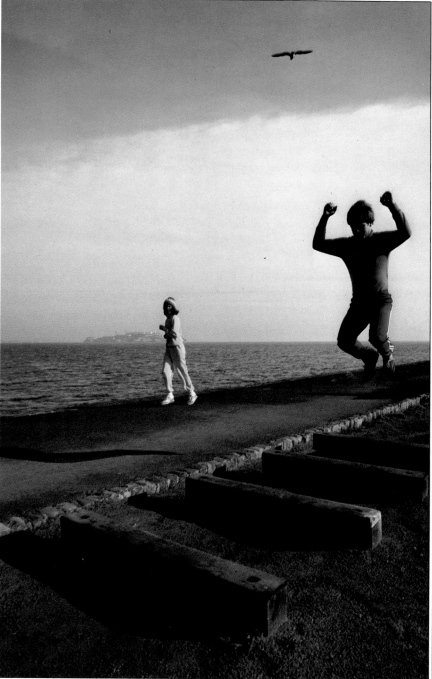

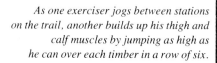

As one exerciser jogs between stations on the trail, another builds up his thigh and calf muscles by jumping as high as he can over each timber in a row of six.

terol. David Doroff, a New York psychologist, was such a case. Active all his life, Doroff took up jogging at the age of 49, quickly built up his stamina and, after running 18 miles with no difficulty, decided to enter the New York Marathon. Just to be sure that he could safely compete, he took a stress test. It showed nothing abnormal. Yet less than a week later, Doroff collapsed at his desk and died. An autopsy revealed that two of his main coronary arteries were 90 per cent blocked and that blood flow through the third was only 40 per cent of normal.

Doroff's case is unusual, but it is not unique. Researchers have tried unsuccessfully to find distinctions that will identify people who, although cleared for exercise by tests, still may be endangered by vigorous activity. There seems to be no common characteristic. Some people who died while exercising or shortly afterward were young. Others were middle-aged. They may have taken up exercise only a few weeks earlier, or they may have been active for years. For many of the victims, the underlying cause of death was undetected coronary artery disease. In some of them exercise precipitated fatal attacks—but it may also have forestalled or minimized earlier episodes.

Despite these drawbacks, the stress test remains the best technique for determining how much exercise is advisable—and for warning when it should be avoided. The clear consensus is that those with obvious heart risks should have a stress test. And a number of physicians think the test is worthwhile if you are over 35 or if you are younger but fit a so-called coronary-prone pattern: if you are overweight, have high blood pressure or elevated blood fats, smoke cigarettes or have a family history of early heart disease.

The warm-up

When you have satisfied yourself—or your doctor—that you can exercise safely, begin to do so slowly. No matter what exercise you have settled on, precede every exercise period by a warm-up of at least five minutes; some exercisers prefer to extend their warm-up session to 10 minutes. This preparation will keep you from placing sudden stresses on your circulatory system, and at the same time it eases joints and stretches muscles to help forestall injuries or soreness.

Exercising muscles makes them contract and sometimes get shorter. Short, tight muscles are more likely than loose, flexible ones to be injured. Warming up counters this effect by increasing the blood supply to the muscles and raising their temperature, making them more pliable and causing them to stretch. Moreover, the chemical reactions that occur inside muscles and power them are abetted by warm muscles and hindered by cold ones.

You can warm up simply by doing whatever form of exercise you have chosen, only more slowly at first. For example, if you plan to run, you can start out by walking five minutes or so, then go into a slow jog for another five minutes, and then increase speed. Such a warm-up helps stretch muscles to some extent, but a series of deliberate stretching exercises (pages 92-97) helps even more. Thus the best warm-up includes two stages.

Stage 1 involves stretching the muscles of the arms, legs and torso slowly. The key word is "slowly." Gradually stretch each muscle to the point where you can feel the strain, but stop before it hurts. Hold the position from 10 to 30 seconds, then relax. Repeat the exercise at least three times. Do not succumb to the temptation to thrust against your muscles to stretch them. Bouncing up and down to touch your toes, for example, can make it harder to reach them. Sudden, jerky movements evoke resistance from muscles. In this case, bouncing can actually shorten the thighs' hamstring muscles—the muscles that toe touching is intended to stretch—or it may even cause a painful tear in the muscle fiber. As you stretch your muscles, a sensation of warmth suffuses them, tangible evidence that you are achieving the desired increase in blood supply.

Stage 2 of your warm-up should be your main form of exercise, done more gently. This gradual approach enables your body to adapt to strenuous activity, warms up the exercising muscles even more and gets the blood flowing faster through your heart muscle, perhaps the most important feature of the warm-up. A plentiful supply of blood to the heart is necessary so that it can meet the muscles' increased demand for blood during exercise. Your heart needs this prepa-

On a trail in New York City, members of a club called the New York Walkers display the gait of competitive race walking—arms pumping across the chest, knees locking with each step, and at least one foot touching the ground at all times. Fast gaining popularity as an exercise, race walking offers the same cardiovascular fitness benefits as jogging, with less risk of injury.

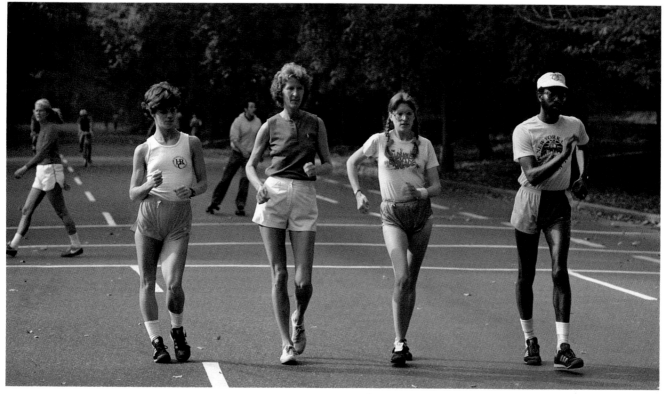

ration for exercising regardless of how fit you are. Stress tests given to athletes before they warmed up revealed heartbeat irregularities that did not appear in tests that followed a warm-up period.

The cool-down

When you have completed your exercise, you should go through the reverse of a warm-up. Do not stop abruptly. Follow exercise with a cool-down period. Walk for 5 or 10 minutes or just keep doing what you were doing, but at a slower rate. Continue your cool-down until your breathing has returned to normal and your heartbeat has slowed.

You may be tempted to skip the cool-down. But doing so can be harmful. During strenuous exercise the blood vessels are dilated so that they can deliver a maximum volume of blood to your muscles. If you suddenly stop exercising, your

heart rate drops and so does your blood pressure. Blood, instead of returning to the heart, tends to pool temporarily in the enlarged veins of the muscles. This accumulation can leave less blood to circulate to the brain, heart and intestine. If the brain does not receive an adequate supply of blood, you may become dizzy or even faint. If your heart does not get enough blood, your heartbeat can become irregular. If your intestine receives too little blood, you may become nauseated.

Warming up and cooling down are the essential beginning and end to every exercise session, regulating the transition between activity and inactivity. A consciously measured level of activity is necessary, too. When you begin to exercise you obviously cannot perform the routines as vigorously or as long as you can after you have been doing them for some time. In addition, the maximum level recommended varies with the individual, depending not only on the kind of exercise performed but also on the age and physical condition of the exerciser.

Pacing exercises for the heart

The vital endurance exercises—running, swimming and bicycling—that build up heart and lungs require particularly careful regulation. They achieve their goal only if you press yourself to work harder than you ordinarily might. Yet some people press themselves too hard, overtaxing the heart and skeletal muscles and causing more harm than good. To pace yourself so that you get the most from your efforts and avoid excess strain, you need only learn to take your own pulse. Then, from the rate at which your heart beats, you can tell how much you are exerting yourself.

Each person's heart has a maximum rate that it cannot exceed, no matter what exercise demands are placed upon it. Several factors limit maximum heart rate, but the main influence is age; the older you are, the slower your maximum heart rate. The greatest benefits come to those people who are able to exercise vigorously enough to raise their heartbeats to at least 70 per cent of the maximum. On the other hand, exercising so hard that the heartbeat exceeds 85 per cent of its maximum rate quickly causes exhaustion without improving fitness noticeably sooner than if the pulse remains slightly slower. This 70-to-85 per cent range in pulse rate, called the target zone, sets the desired pace of endurance exercises for most people.

To find your target zone, of course, you must determine your own maximum heart rate. It can be measured precisely during a stress test, but it can also be approximated accurately enough for exercise purposes by subtracting your age from the number 220. A person 35 years old, for example, has a maximum heart rate of about 185 beats per minute; his target zone is 130 beats per minute (70 per cent of 185) to 157 beats per minute (85 per cent of 185).

When you are not exercising—relaxing in a chair—your heart pumps at about 40 per cent of its maximum rate; if you get up to answer the telephone, the rate may rise to more than half the maximum.

Using your target zone to gauge effort

Aerobic exercise for your circulation and respiration is meant to make your heart work harder than it usually does. How much harder you should make it work is a critical question. If you do not exercise vigorously enough, your fitness will improve at a frustratingly slow rate. Overstrenuous exercise, however, will not substantially improve the speed at which you progress; worse, it will cause unnecessary discomfort—the reason that many people have for giving up exercise—and may strain your heart enough to trigger a heart attack.

To see if you are exercising too hard (or not hard enough) stop briefly from time to time and determine your heart's rate of operation by taking your pulse (page 39). To make sure that the exercise is both effective and safe, step it up or slow it down as needed to keep your pulse rate within a range known as the target zone. Your own target zone is determined by your age; as you get older, the top and bottom of your target are marked by progressively lower pulse rates (below). But the speed at which you must walk, run or bicycle to reach it depends on how fit you are. People in poor condition can usually get their pulse rates into the target zone with a brisk walk; fit individuals must exercise more vigorously.

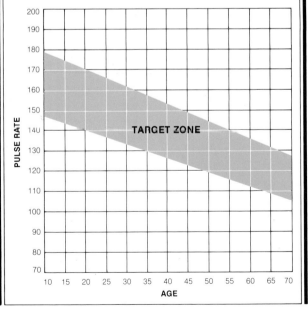

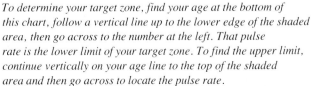
To determine your target zone, find your age at the bottom of this chart, follow a vertical line up to the lower edge of the shaded area, then go across to the number at the left. That pulse rate is the lower limit of your target zone. To find the upper limit, continue vertically on your age line to the top of the shaded area and then go across to locate the pulse rate.

Because such minor changes in the level of activity cause relatively large changes in heart rate, you must check your pulse frequently during exercise if you are to keep within your target zone. If your heart rate falls below the target zone, exercise a little more vigorously; if it creeps above, slow down a little. To see if you are in your target zone, stop exercising briefly. As quickly as you can, put two fingers of either hand along one side of your esophagus below the jawbone and press them gently back toward the large neck muscle. You should feel the beating pulse of your carotid artery, a large vessel that supplies blood to the brain. With a little practice you can learn to do this quickly and easily. Count your pulse for exactly 10 seconds and multiply by 6 to find the number of beats per minute. Do not count for more than 10 seconds; your pulse slows down so fast when you stop exercising that you will get a falsely low reading if you count your pulse any longer.

With a little practice, you will be able to tell when you are in the target zone, even without stopping to count your pulse. This is one simple clue for most people, according to David Costill, Director of the Human Performance Laboratory at Ball State University in Indiana: "If you can't talk while you're exercising, you're working too hard."

If you are able to raise your pulse into the target zone, try to keep it there for at least 20 minutes and preferably for 30 minutes. For best results do this three times a week with no less than one day or more than two days between exercise sessions—Tuesday, Thursday and Saturday or Sunday, for example. More exercise than this is unnecessary for the beginner; it brings little additional benefit, and—unless you have been exercising for at least two or three months—it can even overstress your body.

This prescription disagrees with the advice of some experts, who promise fitness with far less exercise. Most researchers who have measured the progress of exercisers maintain that a weekly regimen of three exercise sessions, each of which keeps your pulse in the target zone for at least 20 minutes, is necessary. With less sustained effort, you may not achieve any noticeable benefits for your heart unless you are in poor condition.

Although most people can exercise vigorously and continuously for as long as 20 minutes at the outset, not everyone will be able to do so or even to bring his heartbeat into the target zone briefly. In that case a slower pace is necessary at the beginning, regulated by Costill's gauge of the ability to talk. This beginning pace generally increases after a few weeks of regular exercise, until at least 20 minutes of continuous exercise within the target zone is feasible.

For most people, six months of such exercise, performed diligently three times a week, improves fitness gradually to the point where performance on the step test rises into the "good" range, a commendable degree of fitness for everyone but competing athletes. Of course, as you become more and more fit, you will expend more energy to keep your pulse in the target zone. But the added exertion will seem no more strenuous than when you first began exercising, proof that you have strengthened your heart and the muscles you use to exercise it.

To maintain this level of fitness, you must maintain the level of exercise that achieved it—20 to 30 minutes of target-zone heart effort three times a week. Slacking off will bring an immediate loss in condition. Conversely, increasing the exercise with longer periods of activity or more frequent ones—as many exercise enthusiasts are tempted to do—will not add as much to the stamina of the heart and lungs as might be expected. Doubling the amount of exercise will not double its effects. Indeed, intensified efforts may cause sleeplessness or chronically sore muscles—symptoms of muscles that have not recovered fully from earlier workouts.

Choosing an endurance exercise

"Of all exercises," Thomas Jefferson once noted, "walking is the best." Many authorities today agree that, of the variety of activities contributing to strong heart and lungs, walking is the first choice, particularly as a start. It is the most popular exercise. You can walk almost anywhere at any time. Speed can be regulated between an undemanding stroll and a brisk pace of nearly five miles per hour to accommodate the target zones of people who differ widely in fitness and age. Walking does not jar your ankles, knees or hips, yet

The hazards of heat and cold

Either hot or cold weather can be dangerous when you exercise outdoors. On a hot and humid day, your body may not be able to dissipate all the heat that vigorous exertion produces, and body temperature may rise until you risk heatstroke. A windy winter day can be so cold that heat drains away from your body faster than it can be replaced; at these times, the risk you run is that of frozen skin, or frostbite.

To gauge the dangers of hot weather *(below, left)*, you must know the outdoor temperature and relative humidity. To use the cold-weather chart *(below, right)*, you need to know not only the temperature but how hard the wind is blowing.

In most cities, you can get these figures through the telephone company's weather-report number, from commercial radio broadcasts or over the government's special weather radio. Or check the temperature with a thermometer, the humidity with an inexpen-

sive instrument called a hygrometer, and the wind with a wind-speed gauge, all available at hardware stores.

With these weather data, you can use the charts to tell you whether it is safe to exercise. In the ''safe'' zone of the heat-and-humidity chart, you can probably exercise without risk. In the ''caution'' zone, it is generally safe to exercise lightly if you drink 16 ounces of water before you start, eight ounces every 15 minutes during your workout and eight ounces afterward, whether you are thirsty or not. When the temperature-humidity combination is in the ''danger'' zone, it is unsafe to exercise at all.

On the cold chart, frostbite is unlikely in the ''safe'' zone as long as your skin is dry. But if your skin is damp—from precipitation or perspiration—cover it, especially that of extremities. In the ''caution'' zone, cover exposed skin even if it is dry. Even protected skin can freeze in the ''danger'' zone; stay indoors.

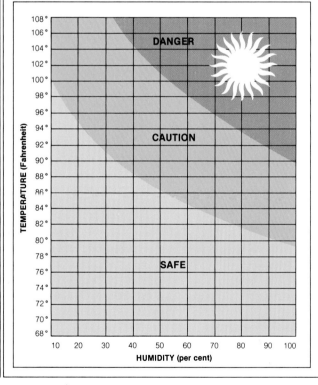

WHEN IS IT TOO HOT?
To determine the risk of exercising in the heat, find the temperature at the left of the chart, then read from it across to the right and stop at the vertical line that represents the relative humidity. On a 90° F. day, for example, if the humidity is less than 30 per cent, the weather is in the safe zone.

WHEN IS IT TOO COLD?
To assess the risk of frostbite, find the temperature at the left of the chart, then add the speed of the wind to your speed when exercising and find this total air speed at the bottom of the chart. The point at which the temperature line meets the total air speed determines whether it is safe to exercise.

it flexes them continuously and rhythmically, both necessary for building stamina.

To begin walking for exercise, first warm up by stretching the muscles of your lower back and the backs of your legs *(pages 96-97)*. If you are able, set out immediately at a pace that will raise your pulse into the target zone. But if your performance on the step test was fair or poor, start much more slowly and gradually. First try to walk a mile continuously at the fastest pace that you find comfortable. If it takes half an hour, you are walking at the rate of two miles an hour. At this rate your heart probably will not reach the target zone. Continue on alternate days to walk a bit faster, increasing your pace each time and checking to see if you are reaching the target zone. After a relatively few sessions, you will find that you can go faster and cover the mile more easily. By the time you can complete a mile in 15 or 20 minutes, your pulse will probably be in the target zone, and you can increase or decrease your cadence to keep your heart beating at the appropriate rate.

If you try for a regular cadence, rather than a constant speed, you will have a gauge of exertion that compensates for walking up hills or against the wind. In other words, slow down when climbing a hill, not by taking fewer steps per minute, but by taking shorter ones. As the weeks pass you will have to step up your cadence to keep your pulse in the target zone. Some people experience a steady improvement; others reach plateaus that last as long as two weeks, then the cadence jumps several steps per minute. In either case, you never go backward, and after four to six weeks you will have to walk noticeably faster to reach your target zone. Within 12 to 14 weeks of regular exercise, you can expect to have raised yourself at least one full level of fitness in the step test.

After three months of walking diligently, almost everyone will have worked up to a cadence of 130 to 140 steps per minute. But to reach the "good" level of aerobic fitness, many people would have to walk even faster. Their cadence would have to exceed 150 steps per minute, a pace so fast that walking becomes uncomfortable.

At this juncture, you can apply various stratagems to slow the cadence of walking while maintaining an effort that keeps your heart in the target zone: Walk in hilly terrain or in loose sand at the beach, or load yourself with extra weight. Most people who must walk very fast to reach their target zones stop walking and start jogging. A jog is a slow run. The heels strike the ground before the toes, as in walking, and not after, as in sprinting, but the legs and arms move faster and more rhythmically than in walking. To jog, take strides of a comfortable length, keep your torso vertical and hold your hands about waist level.

Unlike walking, jogging requires special equipment: a pair of shoes to cushion your ankles, knees, hips and back against the jolts caused as your feet strike the ground. Jogging shoes are expensive compared with garden-variety sneakers, but you really cannot manage without them. Sneakers, for example, are too stiff in the sole, too low in the heel and too weak along the sides to support your foot for jogging, and if you wear them you can injure your feet. Almost any manufacturer's jogging shoe will do if it can pass the tests described on page 77.

Some attention should also be paid to clothes for walking or jogging, although specially designed outfits are not necessary. In summer, when the object is to keep as cool as possible, shorts and a T-shirt are ideal. For jogging, but not necessarily for walking, a man may be more comfortable wearing an athletic supporter. A woman with full breasts may want to buy a support bra especially made for joggers.

Even comfortable clothing may not keep you cool if you exercise in the heat of summer. Hot weather causes your heart to beat faster than it would during the same exercise on a cooler day—it must work harder to supply more blood to the skin so that internal heat is dissipated more efficiently—and you will feel hotter inside than you normally do. But after a couple of weeks, your body will adapt to exercising in the heat. Your pulse rate will fall and your body will increase perspiration to keep you cooler.

Nevertheless, some days are so hot and humid that your body cannot cool itself adequately even though you perspire freely. Postpone your exercise if the combination of temperature and humidity falls in the danger zone on the chart on page 74. Under such conditions body temperature can rise to

Choosing the right jogging shoe

If you jog for exercise, the one indispensable item of equipment is a pair of sturdy running shoes. Each time your foot strikes the ground—about 800 times a mile for each foot—it experiences a jolt that travels up through your leg to the small of your back; the impact can damage tendons or the bones in your legs and feet. Only shoes that are designed especially for running can stave off aches and pains.

Selecting the proper shoe involves a process of elimination—one manufacturer offered more than 40 models in one of its catalogues. Before trying on any running shoe, examine it to make certain that it is built like the one below. Also, check the sole to see that it is suitable for the surface that you plan to run on *(opposite, top right)*, that it flexes properly and that the back of the shoe, or heel counter, is stiff enough to hold your heel in position as you

run *(opposite, bottom)*. Then try on the shoes. For the best fit, wear the same kind of socks you use for running, and tie the laces yourself—salesmen often pull them too tight.

The shoe should fit snugly from the ball of your foot back to your heel. But your toes should have plenty of room *(opposite, top left)*. The heels should feel resilient but not mushy. If the heel seems to lose its resilience under your weight, look for another shoe with firmer cushioning.

A pair of shoes chosen in this way should last for about 1,000 miles of running before the interiors of the soles succumb to the constant pounding and no longer cushion your feet. Thus, if you jog three times a week for half an hour at a moderate speed of six miles per hour, you can expect a good pair of shoes to last nearly two years.

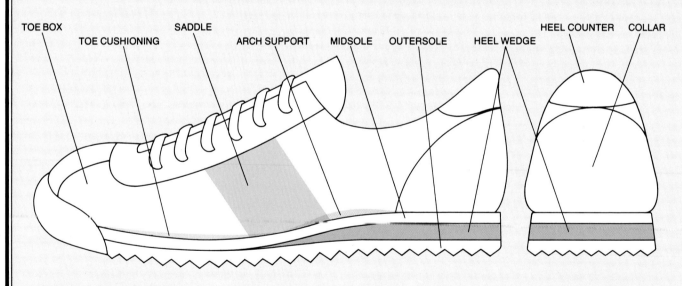

TOE BOX TOE CUSHIONING SADDLE ARCH SUPPORT MIDSOLE OUTERSOLE HEEL WEDGE HEEL COUNTER COLLAR

ANATOMY OF A RUNNING SHOE
The toe box of a running shoe should be roomy, letting your toes move freely to prevent blisters, corns and bruising beneath the toenails. A reinforced saddle, usually strengthened with boldly colored leather, holds the middle of your foot in place. At the back of the shoe, a stiff heel counter, topped with a flexible collar to prevent chafing, keeps your heel from slipping to the side.

Inside the shoe, beneath an innersole, lie the soft arch support and cushioning for the toes. Outside the shoe, under the toe, a midsole of spongy plastic is laminated to an outersole of durable rubber. But under the heel, which must absorb the greatest shock, the midsole is thickened or the two soles are separated by a spongy plastic heel wedge to provide extra cushioning.

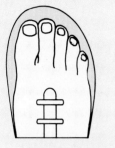 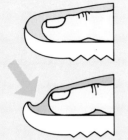

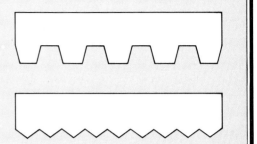

THE FIT AT THE FRONT

When trying on the shoe, be certain there is enough room for your toes at the sides and front (above, left), as well as at the top (top right), so that these parts of the shoe do not put pressure on your toes. To make sure you have enough room in front of your toes, press your thumb across the tip of the shoe (bottom right); the fit is correct if your thumb does not overlap your longest toe.

DIFFERENT TREADS FOR DIFFERENT RUNNERS

A waffle-patterned tread on the outersole (top), suitable for anyone who runs on pavement, emphasizes cushioning over durability. A shallower tread (bottom), longer wearing but not as shock absorbent, is better for running on softer surfaces.

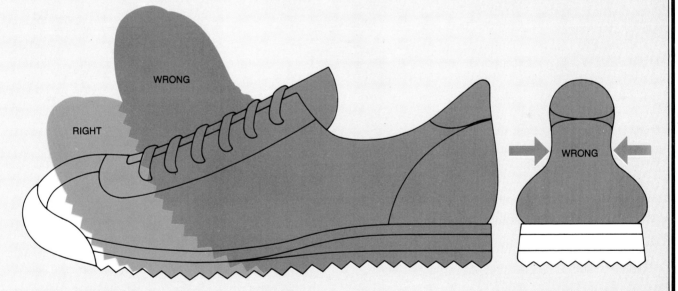

CHECKING STURDINESS

Two quick tests help determine whether a shoe is built to hold your foot securely as you land on it with a force at least twice your weight. First, hold the shoe at either end and flex the sole (above, left). It should bend readily where the ball of your foot would go (yellow); a shoe that bends farther back (red) will not give you enough arch support, and a poorly supported arch can lead to the pain of runner's knee (pages 136-137). Next, with the thumb and fingers of one hand, squeeze the sides of the heel counter (above, right). It should feel firm. If the heel counter collapses easily under such pressure (red), it will allow your heel to slip sideways in the shoe, beyond the edges of the sole; this will place undue strain on your ankles, legs and knees.

well over 100° F. and precipitate a dangerous heatstroke from excessive loss of water through perspiration. To fend off the effects of the heat, drink a glass of water or other liquid, not ice-cold, about 15 minutes before you begin exercising, another one halfway through your 30-minute session and a third after cooling down. If you exercise more than half an hour, drink a glass of water every 15 minutes. If in spite of precautions you notice symptoms of heat exhaustion (headache, unsteadiness, nausea or clammy skin) or of dangerous heatstroke (a feverish feeling and hot, dry skin), begin your cool-down period immediately. If possible, cool down in shade, even if you must walk in circles under a tree. Drink your fill of cool liquids; the body absorbs them faster than it does warm ones.

During spring, fall and winter, the possibility of overheating is remote. But exercising in extreme cold presents a different hazard—frostbite, particularly on windy days. On a zero day, for example, a wind of 20 miles per hour has the effect—known as the wind-chill factor—of lowering the temperature to –39° F., cold enough to begin freezing exposed flesh within one minute. To avoid frostbite, wear gloves and a ski mask or a combination of garments to cover your head, face and ears whenever the combination of temperature and wind speed drops into the danger zone in the frostbite chart on page 74.

Except to provide protection against frostbite, you do not need as much clothing for winter exercise as you might expect. On even the coldest days, all that most people need to be comfortable are long underwear under loosely fitting pants and a sweater under a lightweight windbreaker. If you are still cold, wear more layers of clothing, not heavier garments. Layers trap heat better and can be shed one at a time as you become warmer.

The hazards of cold and heat (and aggressively vigilant dogs) are not everyday problems for walkers and joggers. More common are sore muscles and stiff joints. They generally can be prevented from causing trouble by proper warm-up and limitation of the duration and intensity of exercise.

Beginning walkers are likely to suffer discomfort in their leg muscles but are bothered less by soreness in leg joints, back or shoulders, which inconveniences even veteran joggers. Sore knees are the most common complaint of joggers. They may be caused by running on pavement. Softer shoes or a softer surface—grass or dirt instead of pavement—can help, but long stretches of dirt or grass suitable for running are rare and they are often uneven, increasing the risk of a twisted ankle. A cinder track at a school athletic field is a good choice. However, running in only one direction around a track can make your knees sore; rounding a curve puts more strain on one side of your knees than on the other. The solution is to alternate directions each time you run.

Jogging strengthens the muscles on the backs of your legs more than the ones on the front. This imbalance can also be a source of knee pain. To correct the problem, exercise the muscles on the front of your legs *(page 106)*.

If leg-strengthening exercises do not alleviate the knee pain, slight irregularities in the structure of your foot may be the cause—not only of sore knees but of discomfort in other leg joints or in the lower back or shoulders. If you have flat feet or if your feet overpronate (if your ankle bulges too far inward as you put weight on your feet), flexible arch supports, available at drugstores, sometimes solve the problem. Severe pronation and other troublesome foot shortcomings, such as a big toe shorter than the second toe or a big toe that points toward the little toe, are more complex. They generally require the attention of a podiatrist (a foot specialist) or an orthopedist (a bone and muscle specialist).

Alternatives to jogging

Some people, in spite of all their efforts to banish pain, seem to suffer chronically as joggers, and for them another kind of endurance exercise is a better choice. Bicycling or swimming is just as beneficial as jogging for improving your heart and circulatory system, and either is less likely to cause joint pain than jogging. Both are free of the harsh jolting that characterizes jogging. Swimming does not strain leg muscles or joints, although it may cause some shoulder and arm soreness. Bicycling strengthens the muscles on the front of the leg to balance the strength that the muscles on the backs of the legs acquire in everyday walking; nevertheless, cyclists can also suffer from sore knees if their feet overpronate—arch supports may be the answer.

Bicycling and swimming require the same general procedures as walking or jogging. After warming up, start slowly, then gradually increase your speed until you find a cadence that brings your heart into the target zone. Maintain that rhythm for 30 minutes—less if you become fatigued—then cool down by exercising slowly for several minutes.

If you decide on cycling, any type of bicycle can be used. However, in areas with even moderate hills or stiff winds, a single-speed bicycle requires more strength than is readily mustered by someone beginning an exercise program. Even a gear system with three speeds may not offer a gear ratio low enough for steep hills or a wide enough choice of intermediate gears to match the bicycle to your fitness level when you are climbing hills.

The solution is a 10- or a 12-speed bicycle. The array of gears may seem confusing at first, but they are easy to get used to, as are the low-slung, or dropped, handle bars that come with most such machines. At first these handle bars may cause stiff shoulders and neck, but they eventually make riding more comfortable by making you lean forward so that road shocks are not transmitted along your spine.

This type of bicycle requires careful adjustment of the seat; otherwise, riding may cause sore knees. If the seat is too high, your leg straightens and your knee locks each time you pedal. If the seat is too low, your knees rotate outward. Either situation can make your knees ache. The solution is simple: Adjust the seat height so that with the ball of your foot on the pedal and the pedal at the bottom of its stroke, your leg is almost straight but your knee does not lock. Then ride with the balls of your feet on the pedals.

Special shoes are generally unnecessary for bicycling, particularly if your bicycle has rubber pedals. But metal pedals, which may be shaped so that they concentrate stress along three ridges under the ball of your foot, can reduce circulation to your toes, making them numb. An inexpensive pair of bicycling shoes, which have steel plates in the soles to spread the load across the bottoms of your feet, will usually restore normal circulation.

Other clothing for biking is identical with that for walking or jogging: something comfortable that keeps you warm on chilly days and cool on hot ones. Because of the wind speed you create while cycling—as much as 12 to 15 miles per hour on a calm day—the need to protect yourself against frostbite occurs at higher temperatures than it does for jogging. In summer, however, the breeze helps you to keep cool by evaporating your perspiration at a faster rate. Nevertheless, heatstroke can strike. Drink something cool before, during and after your 30-minute workout so that you do not become dehydrated, and if heatstroke symptoms appear, cool down immediately.

Besides posing a risk of heatstroke, hot weather can also aggravate a peculiar allergy in some people—an allergy to exercise itself. Dr. Albert Sheffer and Dr. Frank Austen, two immunologists at Harvard Medical School, first reported its existence in an article in the August 1980 *Journal of Allergy and Clinical Immunology*. They pointed out that it usually struck practiced exercisers in good condition. Many of them suffered from other allergies or had relatives who did, and the worst attacks occurred on the hottest days.

The allergic reactions that the Harvard immunologists saw customarily began with itching and reddening of the skin during exercise. Hives erupted, and palms, soles and faces began to swell. In the most serious cases the victims developed symptoms identical with those brought on by foods, drugs or insect stings: The exercisers became nauseated and had difficulty breathing; their blood pressures dropped and heartbeats became irregular. Some collapsed in anaphylactic shock, a reaction that can be fatal if not treated promptly. Drs. Sheffer and Austen suggested that an exerciser go immediately to a doctor or a hospital emergency room at the first sign of hives.

One form of exercise that poses few of the risks associated with hot weather is swimming. No matter how hard you swim, the cool water of a pool can draw off all the excess heat that your body can produce. On the other hand, water that is too cold can extract too much heat from your body, causing you to lose consciousness. If your skin turns pink while you are swimming, get out of the water; it is too cold.

Swimming to stay young

The 70-year-old woman was barely out of breath at the end of an hour's steady swimming — 100 laps of a 25-yard pool, more than one and a half miles. "If I didn't swim," said Eva Bein of New York, "I'd be just another old woman. But I feel so young when I swim. A fantasy, perhaps, but it keeps me going." Mrs. Bein's fantasy has more than a little basis in fact. Exercise expert Paul Hutinger of Western Illinois University referred to regular swimming as "the closest thing yet to an anti-aging pill."

Vigorous swimming — fast enough to keep your pulse rate at 70 to 85 per cent of its maximum (*page 72*) for at least 15 to 20 minutes three times a week — is one of the best forms of exercise. It builds arm, shoulder and leg muscles, and provides aerobic conditioning as effectively as jogging. And it does not shock joints and bones, as some land-based exercises do.

Most people intent on conditioning swim laps in a pool with swimming lanes at least 20 yards long. In smaller or crowded pools, the restrained-swimming methods at right are useful; they and the techniques below can also strengthen particular muscles.

PUSHING A KICKBOARD
With your torso kept afloat by a wooden or plastic board, swim using your legs alone. Coaches use kickboards to isolate the mechanics of kicking and to build strength in the legs; the boards also increase the effort required of the heart, which must pump large volumes of blood to the distant leg muscles.

TOWING A PULL BUOY
Hold the buoy — two plastic-foam cylinders linked by a strap — between your legs, with one cylinder at the front of the thighs and the other at the rear; swim with your arms alone. This arm and shoulder exercise calls for less exertion than leg exercises since it requires less blood to be pumped over a shorter distance.

THE STATIONARY FLUTTER KICK
Hold onto the side of the pool and extend your body in a horizontal position. Hold your knees stiff and kick, fluttering the legs, for 20 seconds; rest 20 seconds; then repeat up to eight times. This exercise is not as tricky as swimming with the relatively unstable kickboard, but will condition the legs equally well.

THE STATIONARY CRAWL
Hook your feet to the edge of the pool gutter or the upper rung of a pool ladder, then perform the arm movements of a swimming stroke at the intervals specified for the flutter kick. This exercise is similar to swimming with a pull buoy (opposite), but more strenuous because you are working against greater resistance.

TETHERED SWIMMING
Fasten your waist to a pool ladder with a restraining belt (this can be improvised from a belt and a leash of elastic tubing or shock cord), then perform any swimming stroke. Caution: This is the most strenuous of pool exercises; do not attempt to keep it up for as long as you would swim laps unrestrained.

Walking, running, bicycling and swimming hardly exhaust the ways to condition your heart, though they are among the most popular ones chosen for that purpose. Some people prefer roller skating or jumping rope, cross-country skiing or sculling. You can skip, roll a hoop, chase lizards or even scrub floors, as long as you keep your heartbeat in the target zone for 20 to 30 minutes three times a week.

For the sake of variety, or with a change of season, many people abandon one exercise for another. If you switch exercises, however, you may discover that you cannot perform the new one at the same intensity as you performed the old. An experiment at Queens College in New York City illustrates the point.

Physiologists tested 15 men on a treadmill to determine their running endurance, then asked them to swim for one hour a day three days a week at a strenuous level—between 85 and 95 per cent of their maximum heart rates. After just 10 weeks the researchers noted an 11 per cent increase in endurance as the subjects swam. Yet the same men, when tested again on a treadmill, showed no improvement at all. While the men's hearts had gained the ability to pump more oxygen-carrying blood, the muscles used on the treadmill were not the ones used in swimming, and consequently could not benefit from the extra oxygen that the heart and lungs were able to deliver. If you want to switch exercises, do so gradually, tapering off the old one as you increase your performance in the new one.

Toward a trimmer physique

If you take up an endurance exercise such as swimming, running or cycling, you will hardly be able to avoid getting rid of excess fat—so long as you do not compensate by eating more. If you jog at a pace of only five miles per hour—a speed that most joggers consider slow after about three months of exercise—you burn up about 500 calories per hour (chart, page 47). A pound of fat contains 3,500 calories, or about the number that can be burned up in seven hours of jogging.

As your level of aerobic fitness increases—that is, with improvement in your oxygen consumption or VO₂max—

your body uses more and more of its fat deposits for energy. The evidence for this is indirect. A 1965 experiment with dogs, whose body chemistry resembles that of humans, showed that an animal that ran regularly on a treadmill derived about six times more energy from fat during exercise than an animal not trained on the treadmill.

Such efficiency in fat usage does not seem to be attainable by humans. If you exercise for half an hour three or four times a week, only about half the energy you need for exercise will come from fat. Nevertheless, as long as you do not repay the energy used in exercising by eating more food, you will still lose a pound of fat for each 3,500 calories expended in exercise. Your body uses additional fat after exercising to supply your energy needs for the rest of the day.

You may be tempted to accelerate weight loss by donning a plastic "conditioning suit" while you exercise. Plastic clothing, by preventing perspiration from evaporating, keeps your body hot and forces you to perspire more than you normally would. Wearing such a suit, you can temporarily sweat away a pound or two, but you will regain the weight when you take your first drink of water, as your body replaces the moisture lost to sweating. More important, this practice is dangerous. Exercising in plastic garments, like exercising on an extremely hot and humid day, greatly increases the risk of heatstroke.

Devices such as conditioning suits are unnecessary in any case; fat will disappear without them. And almost as a bonus, the muscles you use to exercise fat away become firmer, changing their shape. Running and bicycling emphasize muscles in the legs. Runners soon acquire sinewy legs that scarcely jiggle; calf muscles and hamstring muscles become particularly firm. Cyclists use the muscles on the front of the thighs and the muscles in the buttocks for most of the power for pushing the pedals. The consequence of these exercises can be powerful-looking legs fitted to a relatively undeveloped torso and arms.

Swimming has a more balanced effect. The various strokes and kicks applied against the constant resistance of the water tend to stress chest, arm and leg muscles in the right proportions to produce an equitably proportioned body.

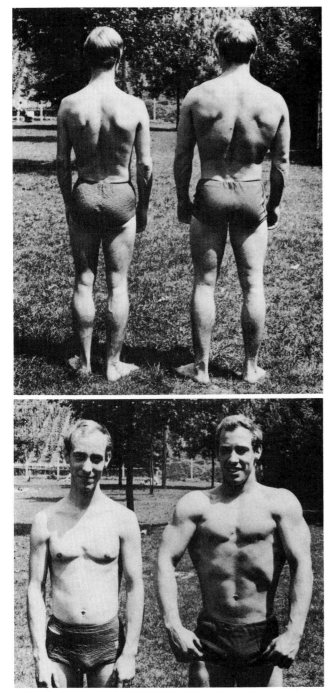

Despite an identical genetic heritage, twin brothers Otto and Ewald Spitz of Germany display startling contrasts in physique, differences produced by differences in exercise. Otto (left), who runs, has a lean build and powerful legs. Ewald, who chose weight lifting, has a barrel chest and a superbly muscled torso and arms—and is about 35 pounds heavier.

If body shaping is a principal goal, exercises other than those undertaken to improve endurance may be necessary. The choice of exercise depends on the part of the body to be shaped—and the extent of the shaping.

Most of this remolding is accomplished by eliminating fat. But firming specific muscles—improving muscle tone—also plays an important role. Dozens of different exercises have been invented to accomplish this wherever tauter muscles are desired *(pages 102-105)*. Sit-ups, for example, are a popular and effective way to help solve the common problem of flab in the middle of the body. They can flatten a sagging, protruding abdomen or slim the hips, depending on how they are done.

Performed with knees locked, sit-ups do more for some hip muscles than they do for the abdomen. Performed with knees bent, they are much more beneficial to the muscles girdling the abdomen. Moreover, there is a technique for performing bent-knee sit-ups that maximizes their stomach-flattening effect. With sit-ups and other exercises you can tone muscles in the chest, arms, abdomen, back, buttocks, hips, thighs and calves. In addition, such exercises can correct posture problems such as curvature of the lower back and rounded shoulders, if they arise because muscles of differing strengths are pulling the skeleton out of alignment. Body-shaping exercises can also, if performed energetically enough, serve as an aerobic program.

Many people undertaking body-shaping routines find that they cannot do some of the more strenuous exercises such as the sit-up. If you cannot complete a sit-up with arms clasped behind your head, as depicted on page 109, try it with your arms crossed on your chest, pressed against your sides or extended above your head. If a sit-up is still too difficult, cheat. Grasp your thighs and use your arms to aid your abdominal muscles in raising your torso. Such self-help may sound counterproductive; indeed, if you never progress beyond the need for it, you will gain nothing in fitness. But more important than achieving form at the outset is training muscles in the full movement expected of them, even if they are too weak to do all the work themselves. After a short period of such training, abdominal muscles become strong enough to pull the body upright without any help from the arms. Even if you can do difficult exercise without resorting to such unorthodoxy, refrain from working yourself to exhaustion, or your muscles will become unnecessarily stiff and sore. Instead, stop when one exercise becomes difficult and go on to another.

If you want to use body-shaping exercises to improve endurance as well, gradually increase to 30 seconds the length of time you can do an exercise, rest for 15 to 20 seconds, then exercise for 30 seconds. By repeating this cycle of exercise relieved by a short break, you can extend the effort of a body-shaping routine so that you keep your pulse in the target zone for 20 to 30 minutes.

This method of improving your ability to repeat an exercise can be carried to extraordinary lengths. In a fitness class conducted by Frank Katch at Queens College in New York, students who could not do a single sit-up when they began were able to perform 200 in one exercise session by the end of the 10-week course.

Exercising for strength

Every exercise in which muscles contract makes them stronger. With aerobic exercise, heart muscle is strengthened so that it can pump a greater volume of blood through your body. The skeletal muscles that you use to perform the exercise—leg muscles in running, for example—become firmer as you exert them to keep your pulse in the target zone. Sit-ups done in search of a trimmer middle strengthen abdominal muscles. In those examples, muscular strength is an incidental benefit of exercise done for some other purpose. You can become stronger faster, however, if you exercise in a way that is designed to promote strength. For fastest progress with least wasted effort, exercise two or three times a week, a schedule similar to one for strengthening your heart or shaping up your body.

Unlike the regimens best suited to endurance and body shaping, the ideal way to build strength is to work muscles near their peak capacity every time you exercise. Between sessions your muscles will recover and become stronger. This strain of intense work or overload on the muscles is necessary to strengthen them, but it can constrict blood vessels and temporarily raise blood pressure during the exercise—especially if the load is heavy and the strain great. It also can aggravate high blood pressure, lower-back pain and hemorrhoids; if you have suffered from any of these disorders or have a heart condition, consult a physician before starting exercises to strengthen muscles.

To exercise muscles until they can do no more work, many people lift weights that are adjustable—the familiar barbell, a rod to which heavy metal disks can be attached. With them, begin exercising with a relatively light stress on your body and increase the load in small increments as you gradually become stronger.

When you start, assemble a load on the barbell that allows you to repeat an exercise 12 times. Because the load you can lift 12 times varies with each exercise, you will have to experiment. Write down the starting weights and use them unchanged for five or six sessions, until you are familiar with the exercises. At the next session, increase the weights—a change of 5 to 10 per cent is about right for most people—so that you can do the exercises only six times; continue using this load during the next several sessions. When you can complete each exercise with the increased load eight times, increase the load again, adding weights so that the number of repetitions again falls to six. Continue this process, adding weights as strength increases.

To get the most out of training with weights, rest for one or two minutes after the first six repetitions, then do six more before going to another exercise. Do a variety of exercises to strengthen your muscles in the full range of motion. Also, think of exercises with weights as having two parts: overcoming gravity to lift the weight and then resisting gravity to lower it. For maximum benefit, do the exercises slowly, taking at least two seconds each time you raise or lower a weight. Slow movements are also safer—the momentum of rapidly moving weights can easily increase until it is more than you can control, and you may not be able to stop a speeding weight before it causes harm.

Weight training is the best way to build muscular strength when a very pronounced effect on very specific muscles is

What to expect from a good health club

Private health clubs have proliferated across North America and Western Europe, and with good reason. The better clubs, like New York City's Cardio-Fitness Center, pictured on the following pages, offer complete programs of exercises tailored to meet individual needs. Fellow members provide enthusiastic support. To the standard gymnasium gear many clubs add ingenious modern exercise machines and such amenities as swimming pools and racquetball or squash courts.

But not all clubs are created equal. If you are considering joining one, examine its facilities and policies before you sign up. Make sure you will be allowed to attend at least four days a week—at your convenience. Inquire about staff credentials; at a top-flight club every instructor has a degree in physical education or exercise physiology. And make certain that a staff member trained to rescue heart attack victims is on duty during club hours.

Tour the exercise room to be sure that the equipment is functioning and that members are supervised by the staff. Finally, visit the club at the time of day you expect to use it. If you hope for speedy sessions during lunch hour, drop by then: The club may be jammed with others who had the same idea.

While workouts begin in the main room of the Cardio-Fitness Center, a new member is tested for the fat content of his body. The calipers are set at several checkpoints to measure fat thicknesses, which are converted to a percentage of body fat. Overweight members gauge their progress by repeated measurements.

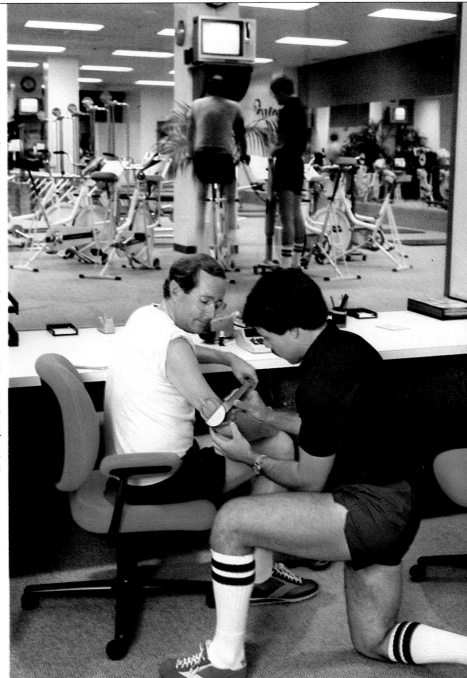

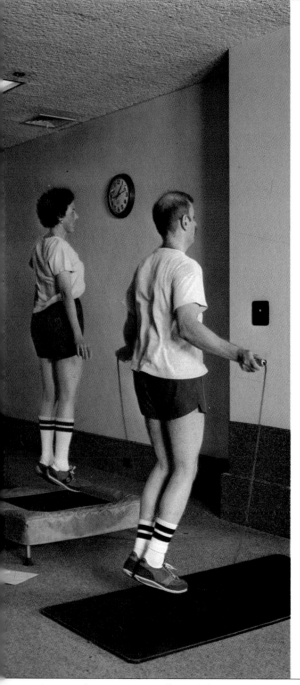

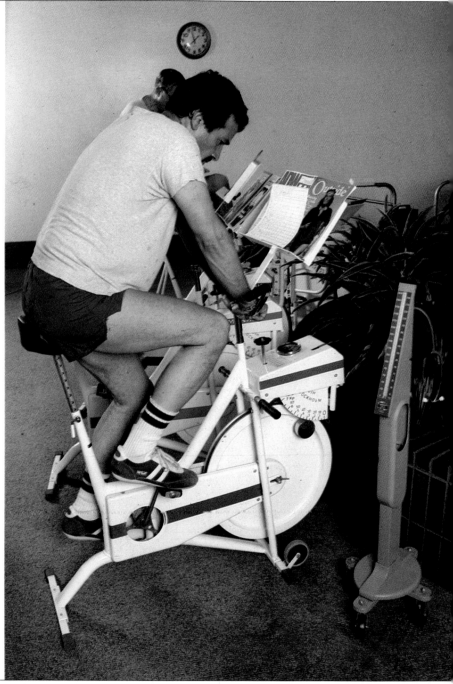

A woman bounces on a small trampoline
while a man skips rope to condition the heart
and improve muscular coordination. Men
and women exercise together at the Cardio-
Fitness Center, which, unlike some
clubs, does not set aside hours for each sex.

As he reviews his program on an exercise chart, this club
member pumps away on a stationary bicycle that can be adjusted
for harder or easier pedaling, depending on the pedaler's
fitness; the machine has a speedometer and an odometer, which
measure the exerciser's "speed" and "distance." The
equipment at right is used for midexercise blood pressure checks.

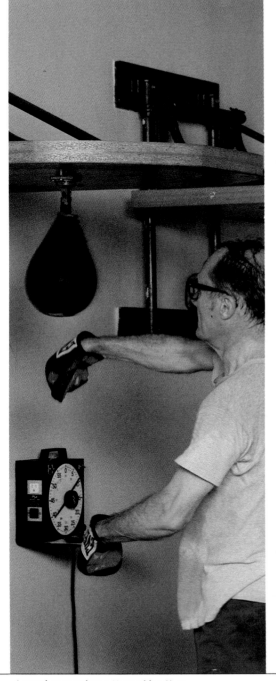

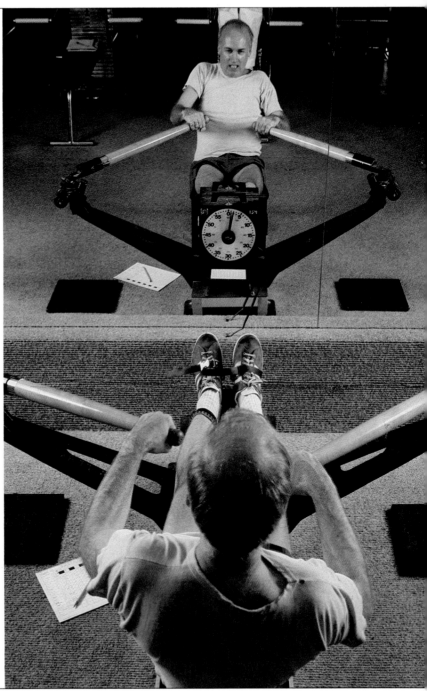

A member punches a ''speed bag'' at the end of his exercise session during a timed cool-down. This period, which also includes dumbbell exercises, allows the speeded-up heartbeat to slow gradually to a level just above normal resting rate.

Feet securely strapped to prevent slipping, a club member watches a clock reflected in the mirror tick off his turn at the oars of a rowing machine. Used both for warm-up and for building endurance, this machine provides one of the few activities that are good for strengthening arms, back and chest as well as building the heart and developing leg muscles.

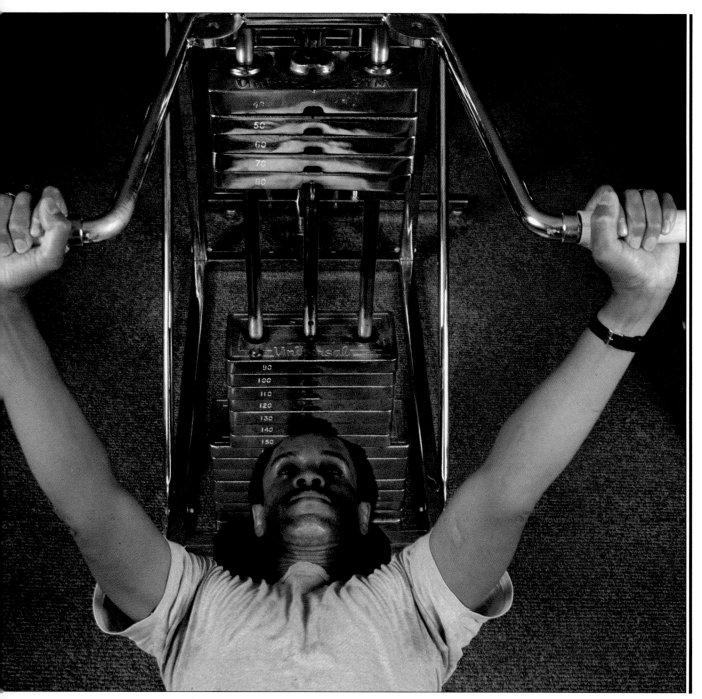

*With his arms fully extended to raise the weights of the modern
machine behind him, a club member performs the movement
known as a bench press. Devices of the kind he is using are much
safer than dumbbells—if he drops the weights, they fall
harmlessly to the stack of weights behind his head.*

desired. It is generally used to correct weakness caused by disease or injury and to develop particular muscles that athletes must use in their sports. But if the goal is simply a general strengthening to aid with the stresses of exercise or everyday chores, an easier method is provided by calisthenics. These old-fashioned activities use the weight of the body itself as the load that helps build the body. Pull-ups to a chinning bar, for example, require you to lift all your weight with arm and shoulder muscles, strengthening them. Push-ups, done by using your arms to raise your body from the floor, strengthen muscles in your shoulders, chest and the backs of your arms *(page 108)*. Abdominal muscles are strengthened by sit-ups *(page 109)*.

Although the effects of calisthenics depend on the load imposed by the weight of your body, that load can be adjusted by variations in the way the exercises are performed. You can make pull-ups easier by supporting part of your weight with your legs; to make them more difficult, add the weight of shoes or other clothing. You can make push-ups easier by raising yourself on your knees instead of your toes, or make them harder by resting your toes on a chair. You can graduate to one-arm push-ups, first on the level and then with your feet raised. Just as you can make sit-ups easier if you help yourself by placing your hands on your thighs, you can make them more difficult by performing them while lying with your head down an incline.

Neither weight training nor calisthenics alone make the best general conditioning or strength-building routine. A better plan assembles the best examples of each type and combines the two into a group of exercises that strengthen all the major muscles in your body.

Because you should mix up exercises in a set sequence to give muscles a chance to recover before you stress them again, it is helpful to set up a series of stations, places where you perform each exercise in the sequence. One man provided eight stations in the confines of a small apartment. The first was for sit-ups, which he did on the bedroom floor with his knees bent and his feet anchored under the bed. Station 2 was a bar in the bathroom doorway for pull-ups. Station 3 was the hallway, where he skipped rope. Then followed

stations for exercising the arms, legs, chest and back with weights. The last station was a five-story stairwell—he walked down from his apartment to ground level, then climbed up again.

How strong you become with a strength-building routine depends on how long you pursue it. One study at the University of Arizona showed that, on the average, after 10 weeks male students increased the maximum load they could lift by 17 per cent, and female students increased their maximum load by 20 per cent.

Exercising tensions away

Almost any exercise is relaxing. Many people report that one of the principal benefits is a feeling of physical and mental ease. For that reason, some prefer to exercise in the evening; the tight shoulders and jumpy nervousness provoked by a difficult day seem to fade, leaving the body relaxed and the mind cleared.

Yet there are often many times during the day when relaxation would be helpful but when it is impractical to take time off for calisthenics or jogging. One method that can be practiced anywhere in 5 or 10 minutes uses consciously directed effort to relax all the muscles in the body. The technique was devised in the early 1900s by Dr. Edmund Jacobson of the Jacobson Clinic in Chicago, Illinois, and became known as progressive relaxation. In succession, groups of muscles are first deliberately tightened, then loosened, until all of them have been relaxed.

The modern adaptation of Dr. Jacobson's technique can be learned fairly quickly, but requires some practice at home. Sitting in a comfortable chair or lying on a bed, close yourself off from distractions. Shut your eyes and hold each group of muscles in your body under tension one at a time for about five seconds. Then allow each one to relax as you focus your attention on the subtle changes in the way that your muscles feel as they become less tense.

You can tense your feet by simply curling your toes. To tense your calves, rotate the top of your foot up and back toward the shin. Lift your legs to feel tension in your thighs and buttocks. To tighten your abdominal muscles, pull in your stomach, then force it out or make it hard. Stress your shoulders and your upper back by throwing your shoulders back as far as you can. Inhale deeply to pull your chest muscles taut, then allow your breath to exhale naturally, neither holding back the air in your lungs nor forcing it out. Lower your chin against your chest to tense your neck muscles. Flex your biceps to tense your arms. And finally, tighten your facial muscles by frowning, squinting and pursing your lips. Use these actions to tense and relax each of the muscle groups at least twice.

The first trial of this method may take as much as an hour or more, but after some practice you will find that you can decrease the time needed for the tensing part of the procedure; soon you will be able to skip it altogether and simply examine each group of muscles for signs of tension, which you can then relax away. By then, easing tension may be accomplished in a few minutes or so.

Such simple, mentally directed efforts to relax generally work to counteract the tensions of everyday routine. However, muscles can become so tight from sitting hours on end in a car or from repeating monotonous but untaxing sets of movements such as painting that active exercises, designed especially for relaxation *(pages 110-112),* are needed to relieve their tightness.

Sticking with it

Learning exercises—of any type, for any purpose—is easy. Performing them regularly is not. ''I sure would like to get involved in running,'' remarked a corporation executive wistfully to his weekend guests as they returned from a Sunday morning jog, ''but I just don't have the time.'' He is probably right. No one who gets up early, starts work by 8 o'clock, drags to bed early and exhausted, and spends many weekends in the office could find open holes in his schedule waiting to be plugged by exercise. What the executive failed to realize was that his house guests—and most others who exercise regularly—once had no time for it either. They had to make time, sometimes inventively, by combining exercise with another activity, and sometimes ruthlessly, by sacrificing a favorite pastime for push-ups.

One of the best opportunities to fit your exercise into a schedule arises on the way to work in the morning and home in the evening. If you live within four miles of your job, it is practical to walk to work; you can do it in an hour or less. Bicycling is practical for distances up to 10 miles or more. Some people even jog to work, if they have a place to shower when they arrive and can carry their clothes in a lightweight knapsack. Others drive partway to work and walk, run or even bicycle the rest of the way.

Combining exercise with commuting to work may not appeal to you. If so, try exercising at times when you feel you would enjoy it most. If that practice fails, try exercising at times when you think you would enjoy it least. Some people who hate to get up early discover to their surprise that a before-breakfast workout makes them energetic throughout the morning. Others who normally feel exhausted after a day on the job feel more refreshed by exercise before dinner than by a nap. Varying the time when you exercise can also help; it keeps exercise from becoming drudgery, something that you are obliged to do.

To exercise three times a week, week after week—as is necessary for lasting benefit—requires not only time but a modicum of discipline as well. Yet it is a rare individual who is sustained in his efforts only by the conviction that what he is doing is good for him. He must also enjoy it. The pleasure of exercise helps explain why joggers exercise in the rain or snow and why people become so enthusiastic about exercise that they fret when forced into inactivity by a severe cold or an injury. Give yourself the best chance to persevere in your pursuit of better fitness; pick an exercise that appeals to you over one that is in vogue as ''the best.''

Some people who find exercise tedious discover ways to divert themselves while doing it. Dr. Grant Gwinup of Irvine, California, had one patient who ''watches television every night,'' he reported, ''while pedaling away on her exercise bicycle. She has a map on the wall and a counter on the bicycle. And she moves a pin every night to show how far she's gone. So far she's traveled from California to the East Coast and up to Canada. Now she's down in South America. I have another lady who doesn't want to go out at night, so

The addicts

For all of its health benefits, exercise—particularly long-distance running—carries a bizarre risk: addiction. After about 30 to 40 minutes or six or seven miles at a stretch, many runners feel a pleasant ''high''; some doctors ascribe it to chemicals automatically produced by the brain to dull the fatigue and pain of a long run. This euphoria can be so enjoyable that runners become dependent on it—in ever-larger doses. In a study of Boston runners who logged at least 75 miles weekly, 24 per cent declared they had changed jobs to make more time for running. Nearly twice as many said their sport had led to a ''major reappraisal'' of their personal relationships.

For a few, the running habit becomes physically destructive—a minor injury can worsen seriously if the addict obstinately refuses to give it time to heal. Recalled one runner who felt pain in his foot: ''I knew something was wrong, but I just could not give up my running. It felt too good; it meant too much; I had to have it.'' Eventually, the man's foot required surgery, and he ran no more.

The casual runner is an unlikely candidate for addiction. But if you are running seven days a week, 10 to 15 miles each day, and if running has become the central concern in your life, it is time to slack off and find alternative exercises.

she walks around her recreation room. She has two TV sets back to back in the middle so she just picks up on one as the other goes out of view.''

Others find that expense and convenience are overriding factors in choosing an exercise that they will stick to. They are certainly two of the reasons for the immense popularity of walking and running. For the modest expense of a pair of jogging shoes, either of these exercises can be pursued practically anytime, at home or away.

Some people find it dreary to exercise alone, preferring the company of others while they get in shape. Organizations exist to bring together groups of people interested in virtually every kind of exercise. Some are volunteer clubs that simply provide companionship. Others sell exercise programs, a place to do them and the guidance of instructors.

Some of these enterprises specialize in specific types of exercise such as stretching routines for flexibility or aerobic dancing—steps set to fast-paced music. Other organizations offer a broader range of activities, including many that require elaborate equipment: weights for strength building, treadmills, exercise bicycles and indoor swimming pools for aerobic exercise, and even courts for racket sports such as tennis and squash. The largest chain of such health clubs in the world, the Young Men's Christian Association, represents a bargain in convenient exercise facilities for almost everyone. Despite the name, you do not have to be young, male or Christian to join. Alternatives to the YMCA in some communities are colleges that offer exercise facilities and classes to the public at reasonable cost.

At the upper end of the price scale reign the private health clubs, where a membership may cost hundreds or thousands of dollars a year. Some people find that the expense itself motivates them to continue exercising. Choosing a health club takes a sharp eye. Most of them glitter on the surface, but underneath they range in quality from superb to abysmal. There are telltale signs to look for and pointed questions to ask (pages 85-88) that will help you determine whether a health club lives up to its name or is just a promoter of get-fit-quick nonsense.

The problems of finding a place—or the motivation—to exercise may be harder for some people than the exercise itself. The solution can arise in an unexpected way. One dramatic example was recounted by Dr. Kenneth Cooper, the former Air Force physician who popularized aerobic exercise. ''A man had angina, a heart pain brought on by even slight exercise,'' said Dr. Cooper. ''Because his angina was so severe, he became depressed and decided to commit suicide by running himself to death. He felt his insurance company would not interpret a running accident as a suicide. So he ran as far as he could until he collapsed of exhaustion. To his amazement, he survived. The next night he ran again and covered a greater distance before he collapsed. Night after night he ran, until he could run two miles without stopping. At this point, his angina disappeared. He became a regular jogger and lost his interest in suicide.''

How to get the most from exercise

Exercises are simple to perform—but not so simple as they may seem. Few people realize, for example, that if you jog to strengthen your heart, your heel should strike the ground before your toes. Running on the toes does not absorb shock as well, and over the distances required for benefit to the circulatory system it creates a high risk of injury.

The pictures on these and the following pages demonstrate step by step the right way to do 39 safe and effective exercises. The exercises were selected from the huge and somewhat daunting repertory used by fitness experts. Which ones you choose depends on what you expect to get out of them.

To help you make up a program of routines tailored to your own needs, the exercises are organized into five groups according to the principal benefit each provides: flexibility, heart conditioning, body shaping, strength and relaxation. Caution: If you suffer from back trouble, heart disease, high blood pressure, asthma, lung disorders or extreme overweight, see your doctor before beginning any exercise program.

Almost all of these exercises can provide the warm-up that is essential before vigorous activity. However, most people prefer to warm up with a simple calisthenics routine such as the stretch demonstrated at right. What follows depends on whether you concentrate on a single goal by performing all the exercises in one group or seek an overall workout by selecting a few from each group.

A BASIC WARM-UP: SIDE-TO-SIDE STRETCH
*Stretch one arm, then the other, straight
up (opposite and center) while you extend
the opposite arm and leg down and out
to the side (below). Repeat six times, holding
each stretch about three seconds.*

Stretching for flexibility

Until recently, stretching exercises generally consisted of fast bounces and jerks, on the theory that the body's momentum would pull kinks out of tight muscles. That approach has proved unnecessary—and even dangerous. Such stretching can strain or tear muscles and tendons, and it often results in postexercise soreness. Slow, sustained stretching, on the other hand, increases flexibility and carries virtually no risk of injury; it has actually been shown to relieve muscle soreness.

For safe stretching do each exercise on pages 92-97 slowly and smoothly until you feel a mild tension in your muscles, then remain motionless. When bending forward, exhale as you begin, then breathe normally as you hold the position. Your muscle tension should diminish slightly within a few seconds; if it does not, or if the stretch becomes painful or cramps your breathing, ease off.

In most stretching exercises the goal is not a lot of repetitions, but long duration of each stretch. In general, hold a stretch for 10 seconds or so at first; after a few weeks, as you become more limber, build up to 30 seconds.

MIDRIFF

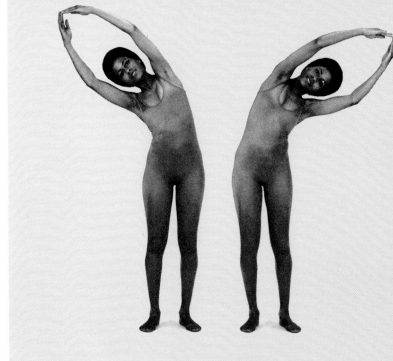

SIDE STRETCH
With your feet 12 inches apart and your arms arched overhead, slowly bend to one side as far as you can and hang there for 10 seconds, letting the weight of your torso stretch your midriff. Stretch to the other side. Caution: Keep your eyes focused on a point directly ahead to maintain balance. At first, stretch each side three times; work up to eight repetitions and longer stretches.

GROIN AND THIGH

GROIN AND THIGH STRETCH
Sit on the floor with your back straight; if you are stiff, sit against a wall. Place the soles of your feet flat against each other, pull them to a comfortable distance from your groin and wrap your hands around your toes (left). Gradually bend forward from the hips, gently resting your arms against your legs for balance, until you feel tension across your inner thighs and groin (below). Caution: Do not bend beyond this point. Hold the stretch 10 seconds, then sit upright; do the exercise three times; after a few weeks, you should be able to do five 30-second stretches.

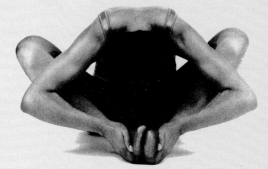

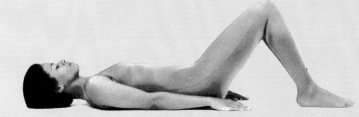

BACK STRETCH (FLATTENED)

*Lie on your back, with your arms alongside your body and resting
on the floor, then bend your knees and rest the soles of your
feet on the floor (above). Lift your knees and pull both shins up
toward your abdomen with your hands, keeping your head,
shoulders and lower back flat against the floor (right). Hold your
legs against your abdomen, at first twice for 10 seconds. Later,
work up to eight times for longer periods.*

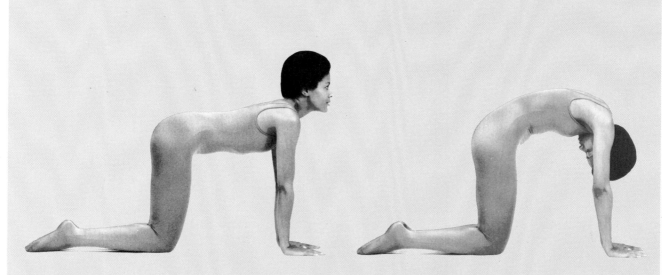

BACK STRETCH (ROUNDED)

*Rest on your hands and knees, with your head in the air (above).
Slowly lower your head, suck in your stomach and round your
back, lifting it as high as you can (right). Hold this position for 10
seconds, then slowly raise your head and return to the initial
position. Do this exercise three times. With practice you should be
able to manage eight repetitions of longer duration.*

HAMSTRING MUSCLE

TOE TOUCH (STANDING)

With feet 12 inches apart, knees straight and arms overhead (near right), lean forward slowly, arms dangling. Caution: If you are stiff, bend your knees slightly. Stop when you feel tension across the backs of your legs, but touch your toes (far right) if you are flexible enough. Hang for 10 seconds, then slowly straighten; gradually work up to five 30-second stretches.

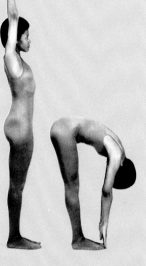

STRETCH (STRADDLE)

Sit on the floor with arms extended to the sides, your legs spread wide and toes pointed up (left, above); if necessary, prop your back against a wall. Keeping your back and legs straight, extend your arms forward and bend from the waist to touch the floor (left, below) or until you feel tension in your groin and the backs of your thighs; hold this position about 10 seconds. The goal is five 30-second stretches.

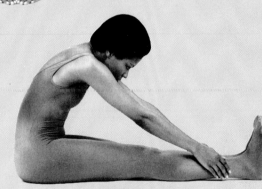

TOE TOUCH (SEATED)

Sit with your legs flat on the floor, heels four inches apart and toes pointed upward, then bend forward from the waist, sliding your hands along your shins and keeping your legs flat against the floor until you feel tension across the backs of your knees and thighs (right, above). If your muscles are flexible enough, extend the stretch to touch your toes (right, below). Hold the position for 10 seconds at first, later for 30 seconds five times.

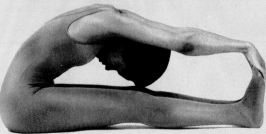

CALF AND ACHILLES TENDON

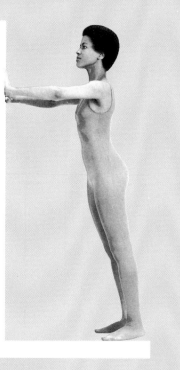

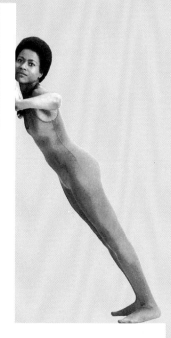

LOWER-LEG STRETCH (WALL)

Stand a little more than an arm's length from a wall, feet pointed forward and flat on the floor, then rest your hands against the wall (far left). Turn your face sideways and slowly lean forward from your ankles— keeping your back straight—until you feel tension in your calves (near left). Hold this position 20 seconds, then slowly push upright with your arms. Start by doing this exercise three times; increase to eight.

LOWER-LEG STRETCH (TABLE)

Rest one leg and heel on a hip-high table; bend the supporting leg an inch at the knee, toes pointed slightly out. (If you are not flexible enough to raise your leg comfortably, rest your calf on a lower support). Slowly bend forward, sliding your hands along the raised leg, until you feel tension along the back of the raised leg (left); if possible, extend the stretch to touch your toes (below). Hold for 10 seconds and repeat the exercise three times with each leg; gradually increase duration to 30 seconds.

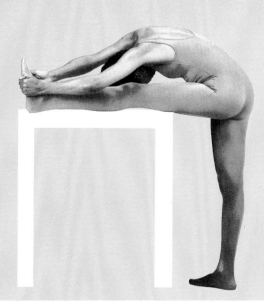

Striding toward fitness

Walking and jogging, two of the best ways of keeping the heart and blood vessels in good shape, may seem a simple matter—as simple, in fact, as putting one foot in front of the other. As fitness exercises, however, both activities are surprisingly intricate.

Before beginning either of these exercises, you should warm up. First, do a combination of the stretching exercises shown on pages 92-97. Then start walking or jogging at an artificially slow pace. After a few minutes of this, your muscles should be loose enough to begin your workout.

After you warm up, getting the most out of walking or jogging depends upon finding the style, pace and distance that are right for you. In establishing each of these factors, compromise between comfort and ease on the one hand, and deliberate exertion on the other.

The style should be the one that you find most natural, maintaining as straight a step and as long a stride as is comfortable. For maximum efficiency, follow the basic rules and avoid the common walking and jogging errors shown here and on pages 100-101.

Good pace is one that falls short of exhausting overexertion. To help you find that point, use a simple ''talk test'' to limit your speed: If you are too breathless to talk while walking or jogging, you are going too fast.

Finding the appropriate distance requires experimenting. For novice walkers, a distance that can be covered in 10 minutes four or five times a week is generally adequate. Later you should be able to walk three miles in 45 minutes; measure the distance with an automobile odometer beforehand or with a pedometer while you are walking.

A beginning jogger is best off alternately walking and jogging for 20 minutes three to five times a week. (If you do your workout on a running track, jog on the straightaways and walk on the turns.) Gradually increase the ratio of jogging to walking; after 8 to 10 weeks, you should be able to jog the full 20 minutes (the build-up may take longer for older persons). Caution: Apply the talk test regularly; if you are breathless, fatigued or uncomfortable, slow down to a walk. After any walking or jogging session, cool down slowly; the easiest way is simply to repeat your warm-up.

THE RIGHT WAY TO WALK
Hold your head high, back straight, and abdomen as flat as possible. Step out at the longest comfortable stride, letting your arms swing loosely at your sides. At each step, land on your heel and roll forward to push off with your toes. Your feet should fall slightly apart, toes pointed straight ahead, as shown in the box below.

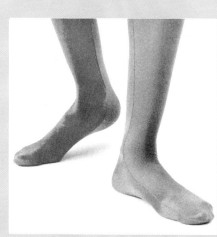

TURNED-OUT TOES

A splayfoot gait, which can injure the arches of the feet and strain ankles, knees, hips and back, can come from sloppy walking habits rather than orthopedic abnormality. Try to correct it by lengthening your stride, which forces your toes to reach forward, pulling your feet more into line. If a longer stride is painful, or if splayfoot persists, consult a foot doctor.

A CROSSOVER WALK

Walking with one foot falling directly in front of the other, a style best reserved for tightrope artists and high-fashion models, produces excessive hip rotation and can cause soreness in the hip joints and the lower back. A lengthened stride and a brisker pace will generally overcome this faulty habit.

TURNED-IN TOES

A pigeon-toed gait can strain the ankles and knees; you may tire easily and find walking painful. The habit may be acquired, rather than caused by a body defect: Try to correct it by stretching your stride and quickening your pace. If this practice proves uncomfortable, or if the habit persists, consult a foot doctor.

JOGGING

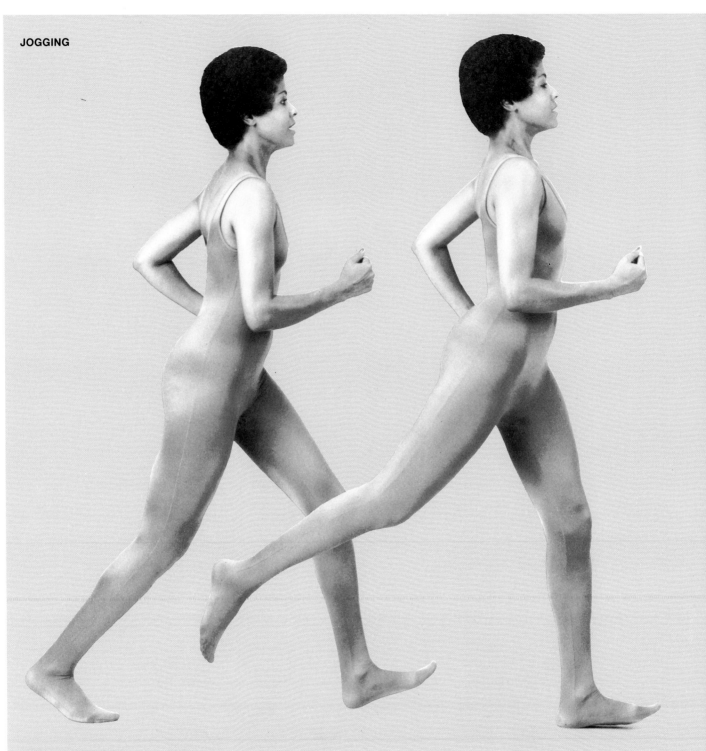

THE RIGHT WAY TO JOG

Keep an upright position, your head high and your arms swinging at hip level; bend your elbows at right angles and hold them three to five inches out from your sides. With each stride, swing your elbows in a straight line. Land on your heels (left) and rock forward to drive off with your toes (right). Keep your stride fairly short; for more exertion, quicken your pace.

COMMON JOGGING ERRORS

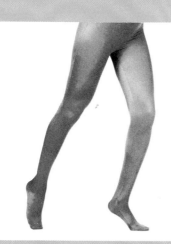

RUNNING ON THE BALLS OF THE FEET
Landing on your toes can cause painful muscle injuries and stress fractures. Cultivate the heel-to-toe stride pictured at left, which distributes stresses along the whole foot; if ''heel and toeing'' is hard for you, run flat-footed.

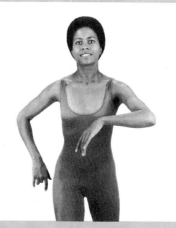

ELBOWS OUT
Pumping your arms from side to side steals momentum. Let your arms swing from your shoulders like pendulums; keep your elbows moving back and forth in a line. Pretend that, as your arm goes forward, you are putting that hand into a hip pocket.

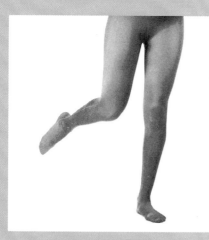

KNOCK-KNEE
This stride dissipates forward momentum. Run with your knees as straight as is comfortable; concentrate on swinging your feet directly beneath your body. Pretend that at each stride your foot is pushing back the ground directly behind you.

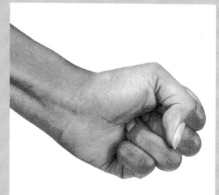

CLENCHED FISTS
Tightly clenched fists tense your arms, shoulders and neck, making you tire easily. Running with open or dangling hands increases muscle tension, too. Cup your hands or close them loosely, with the fingers touching one another lightly.

CALVES

Firming soft spots

Most people seeking a good body shape simply want the body contours to be pleasing to the eye—a reasonable objective, since a pleasing shape is usually a healthy one as well. If a good shape is your goal, remember that no single exercise will give you the overall muscle tone and appearance you are after. You must decide for yourself which muscle groups you need to tone, then select body-shaping exercises for those areas. Whatever exercises you choose, do not neglect posture, which has a profound effect on shape.

Whether you are standing or sitting, hold your head erect, with the profile vertical and the chin level. Keep your back straight but not rigid, your shoulders back but not pinched behind you. Position all your standing weight squarely above both feet, on an imaginary vertical line from the top of your head to a point between your feet; point your toes straight ahead or very slightly outward.

When you are seated, keep your feet on the floor and your hips as far back in the chair as possible; bend from the waist, and do not let your head and shoulders sag forward.

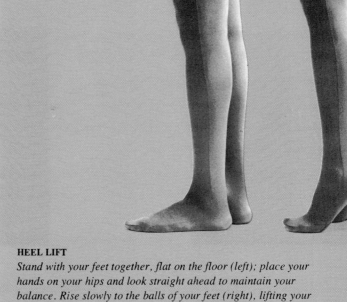

HEEL LIFT
Stand with your feet together, flat on the floor (left); place your hands on your hips and look straight ahead to maintain your balance. Rise slowly to the balls of your feet (right), lifting your heels as high as you can without rocking back and forth; hold this position for five seconds, then slowly lower your heels to the floor. Repeat the exercise 20 times.

HIPS

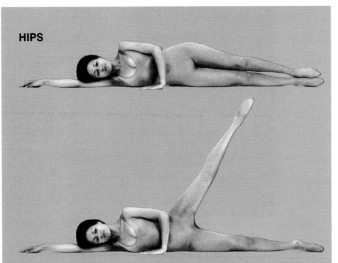

LEG LIFT (SIDE)
Lie on one side, keeping your lower arm extended under your head and your upper arm folded across your waist, with the palm flat on the floor (top). Lift your upper leg vertically as high as you can (bottom)—try to point your toes toward the ceiling—then slowly lower your leg to the floor. Repeat the exercise 15 times on this side. Reverse sides and repeat the sequence.

BUTTOCKS

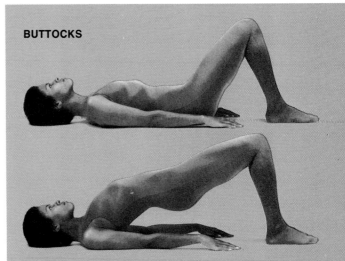

HIP LIFT
Lie on your back with your knees bent, and your arms and feet on the floor (top). Slowly raise your hips, forming a straight line from your shoulders to your knees (bottom), then slowly lower your hips to the floor. Repeat the exercise about 15 times. Caution: This exercise is not recommended for individuals who have problems in the lower back.

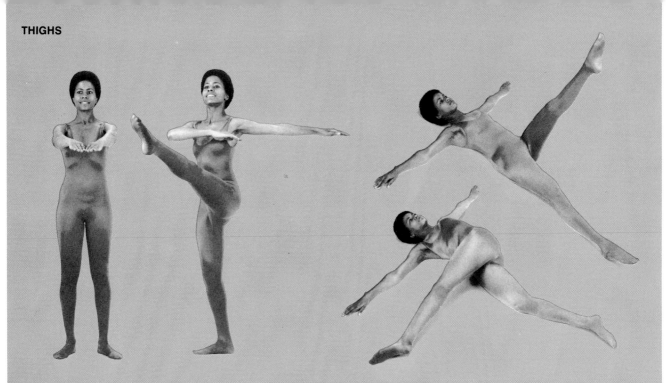

TWIST AND KICK

Stand with your feet about six inches apart and extend your arms forward at shoulder level (left). Then bend your right arm across your chest and thrust your left arm behind you, pulling your torso to the left; at the same time kick your left leg, the toes pointed, up and to the right (right). Return to the starting position, then reverse, twisting your torso to the right and kicking your right leg to the left. Repeat 10 to 15 times with each leg.

TRUNK ROLL

Lie on your back with your arms extended at right angles to your body, palms flat on the floor, then point your toes and raise your left leg as high as you can (top). With your arms still flat on the floor, swing your left leg across your body (bottom); if possible, touch the fingers of your right hand to the toes of your left foot. Return to the starting position and do the exercise with the other leg. Repeat the roll 10 to 15 times with each leg.

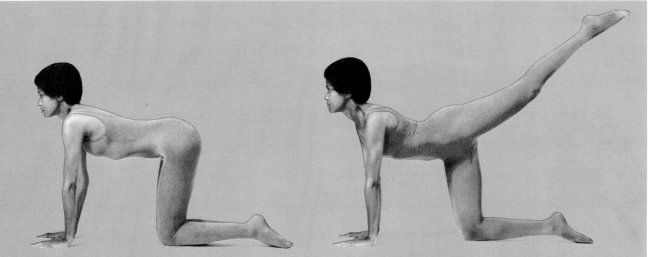

LEG LIFT (KNEELING)

Kneel on all fours, with your back straight and your weight distributed evenly; keep your head up, facing ahead (above). Straighten one leg and point its toes; slowly extend it back and up as high as you can (right). Caution: Do not arch your back to the point of strain. Lower the leg slowly. Repeat about 15 times. Then do the exercise with the other leg.

ABDOMEN

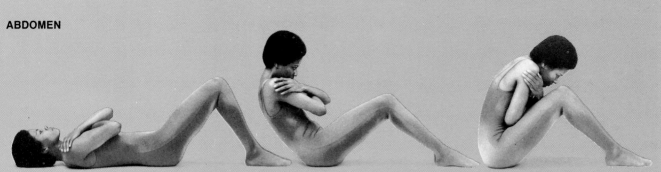

SIT-UP (EASY)
Lie on your back, feet flat on the floor, with your knees bent at 90°
angles and your hands grasping opposite shoulders (left). Curl
your body slowly and smoothly into a sitting position (center and
right). Hold for a few seconds. Roll slowly back to the floor.
Caution: Keep your back rounded throughout. Beginners should
do the exercise three times; the goal is 15 to 20 repetitions.

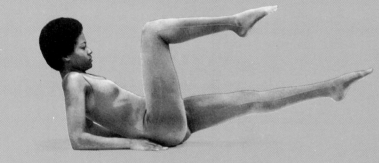

BICYCLE KICK
Sit on the floor, resting your weight on your
elbows and forearms, then raise both legs
slightly and move them in a circular motion,
drawing one leg over your chest while
extending the other leg as far as you can.
Caution: Keep your lower back flat on
the floor. Do 20 revolutions.

FLUTTER KICK
Lie on your back with your hands flat on the
floor, palms down and tucked against
your buttocks; then raise your head and legs
slightly (top). Caution: Keep your
lower back flat on the floor. Keeping legs
straight and toes pointed, move your
legs about four inches straight up and down
in opposite directions (middle and bottom).
Your feet should never touch the floor,
but you can adjust the difficulty of the kick
by altering the distance of your legs from
the floor. Continue for 20 to 30 seconds.

SHOULDERS AND UPPER BACK

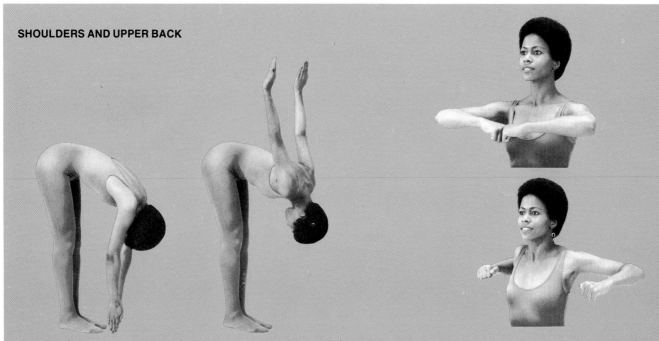

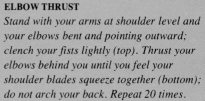

STRAIGHT-ARM LIFT

Stand with your feet together or slightly apart, then bend at the waist, keeping your legs straight and letting your arms dangle (left). Slowly raise your arms behind you, keeping them as straight as possible and bringing them as high as you can (right)—you should feel your shoulder blades pinch together—then lower your arms gradually. Repeat the exercise 10 to 15 times.

ELBOW THRUST

Stand with your arms at shoulder level and your elbows bent and pointing outward; clench your fists lightly (top). Thrust your elbows behind you until you feel your shoulder blades squeeze together (bottom); do not arch your back. Repeat 20 times.

UPPER ARMS

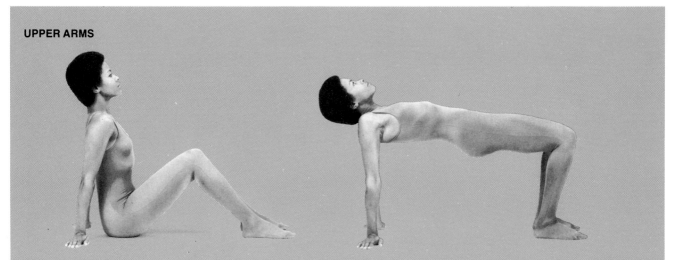

CRAB LIFT

Sit on the floor with knees bent at about a 90° angle, your feet a shoulder's width apart and your fingers on the floor at right angles to your sides (above). Slowly raise your body until it forms a straight line, and hold four seconds (right); do not arch your back. Return to the beginning. Repeat six times. Caution: This exercise is not recommended for anyone with lower-back trouble.

Training for strength

To build stronger muscles, you need not invest in expensive barbell sets or gimmicky devices. Simply exercising against the load provided by the weight of your own body will do the job. Such exercise does not require special equipment, and you will not run the risk of developing a muscle-bound physique.

Each group of muscles must be strengthened separately. To balance your exercise program, you probably will want to exercise several muscle groups; if so, be sure that consecutive exercises tax different muscles. For example, you might follow a hanging knee lift *(page 109),* an exercise for the abdomen, with a session of jumping jacks *(opposite, top),* which strengthen the calves.

To be effective, strengthening exercises should be performed three to five times a week. The benefits of many—especially of knee bends, crossed-leg lifts, push-ups and sit-ups—are increased if you do them at a constant, slow pace from beginning to end. In a push-up *(page 108),* for example, raise yourself from the floor slowly, then lower yourself at an equally slow rate.

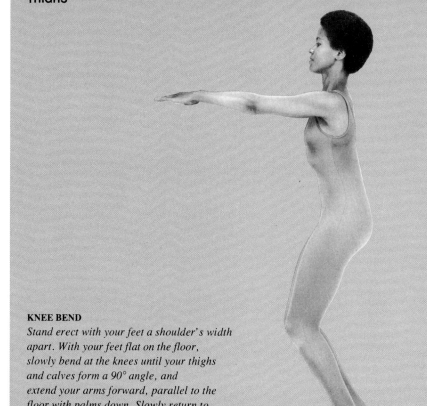

KNEE BEND
Stand erect with your feet a shoulder's width apart. With your feet flat on the floor, slowly bend at the knees until your thighs and calves form a 90° angle, and extend your arms forward, parallel to the floor with palms down. Slowly return to the original position. Caution: Keep your back straight and your head erect; a forward lean can strain your back. Repeat the exercise 10 to 15 times.

THIGHS AND CALVES

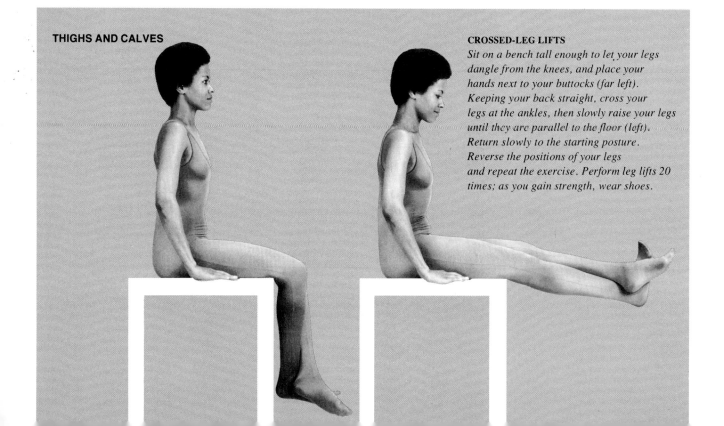

CROSSED-LEG LIFTS
Sit on a bench tall enough to let your legs dangle from the knees, and place your hands next to your buttocks (far left). Keeping your back straight, cross your legs at the ankles, then slowly raise your legs until they are parallel to the floor (left). Return slowly to the starting posture. Reverse the positions of your legs and repeat the exercise. Perform leg lifts 20 times; as you gain strength, wear shoes.

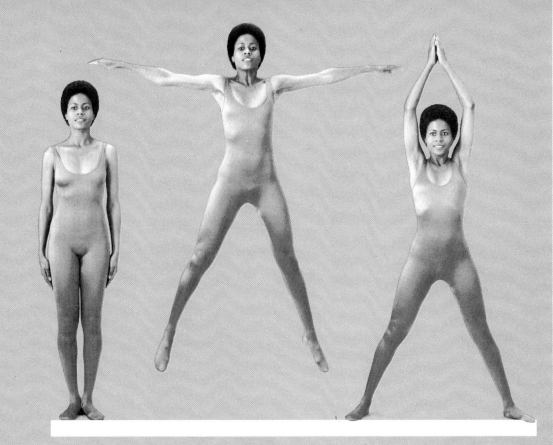

JUMPING JACKS

Stand erect, feet together and arms at your sides (left). Jump up from the floor, swinging arms up and to the sides (center); land with your feet about 24 inches apart, clapping your hands above your head as your feet hit the ground (right). Finally, jump from the floor and return to the starting position. Repeat as vigorously and fast as you can for about one minute.

SQUAT THRUST

Crouch with your hands flat on the floor, holding your head up; resting on the balls of your feet, tuck your left leg under your chest and extend your right leg as far behind you as possible (top). In a bouncing motion, reverse the positions of your legs (bottom). Reverse the legs again to complete the cycle. Start exercising with 12 cycles and work up to 36. Caution: This exercise is strenuous and requires a good sense of balance; begin with care and increase the number of cycles gradually.

SHOULDERS AND CHEST

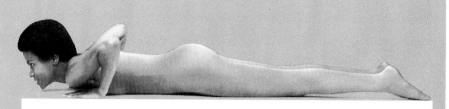

PUSH-UP (EASY)

*Lie on your stomach with your legs together
and your hands under your shoulders,
your fingers pointing straight ahead (top).
Keeping your knees and lower legs on
the floor, raise your upper body until your
elbows lock, forming a straight line from
head to knees (bottom). Slowly lower
yourself. Caution: Breathe normally
throughout this exercise—and stop if you
feel strain. Do the exercise twice; work up
to 10 repetitions. As your strength increases,
do the harder push-up shown below.*

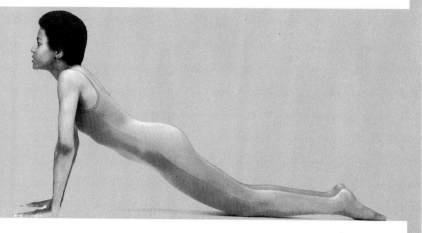

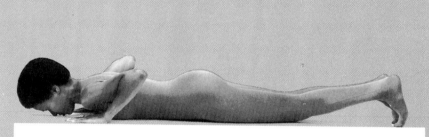

PUSH-UP (ADVANCED)

*Lie face down on the floor, hands tucked
under the shoulders, fingers pointing
straight ahead (top). Keeping your toes on
the floor, raise yourself until your
weight is supported on your hands and toes,
and your body forms a straight line
(bottom). Slowly lower your body to the floor.
Caution: Observe the cautions for the
easy push-up above. Start with four
repetitions, and work up to 20 or more.*

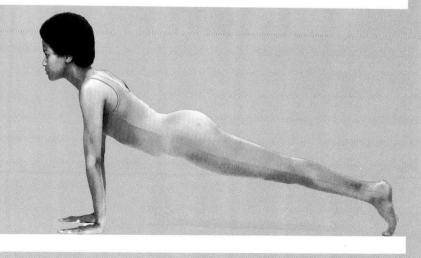

PRIMARY AND SECONDARY BENEFITS OF EXERCISES

The 39 exercises shown on the preceding pages are grouped by their primary benefits, but each has secondary benefits. A sit-up primarily shapes the abdomen but also strengthens it and is a good warm-up. The table lists the exercises alphabetically; a red bar indicates primary purposes, blue secondary.

Legend: Primary benefit (dark) = P, Secondary benefit (light) = S

Exercises	Flexibility	Cardiovascular fitness	Body shaping	Strength	Relaxation	Warm-up
Body tuck	S				P	
Circles, head	S				P	S
Circles, shoulders	S				P	S
Jogging		P				S
Jumping jacks		S		P		S
Kick, bicycle			P	S		
Kick, flutter			P	S		
Knee-bend			S	P		
Lift, crab			P	S		
Lift, heel			P	S		
Lift, hip	S		P			
Lift, knee (hanging)			S	P		
Lift, leg (kneeling)			P	S		S
Lift, leg (seated, legs crossed)			P	S		
Lift, leg (side)			P	S		
Lift, straight-arm			P	S		
Lotus, half (modified)	S				P	
Lotus, half (standard)	S				P	
Push-up (advanced)			S	P		S
Push-up (easy)			S	P		
Roll, trunk (on floor)			P			
Roll, trunk (standing)					P	S
Sit-up (easy)			P	S		
Sit-up (incline board)				P		
Stretch, back (flattened)	P				S	
Stretch, back (rounded)	P					
Stretch, body (on floor)	S				P	
Stretch, groin and thigh	P					S
Stretch, lower leg (table)	P					S
Stretch, lower leg (wall)	P					S
Stretch, side	P					S
Stretch, straddle	P					S
Stretch, warm-up						P
Thrust, elbow	S		P	S		
Thrust, squat		S	S	P		S
Toe touch (seated)	P					
Toe touch (standing)	P					S
Twist and kick			P	S		
Walking		P			S	S

Playing games to stay in shape

The budding science of sports physiology
Which games are good for you
Eating to play better
Building strength for athletics
Flexibility: too tight or too loose?
Treating injuries

In the 12th Century, "futballe"—the precursor of soccer—so distracted Englishmen from compulsory archery practice, which was deemed essential for national defense, that King Henry II prohibited the game. In 1245 the Archbishop of Rouen barred his ecclesiastics from playing court tennis. And in 1314 Edward II of England renewed the ban on soccer, proclaiming that "forasmuch as there is great noise in the city caused by hustling over large balls from which many evils might arise which God forbid; we forbid, on pain of imprisonment, such game to be used in the city."

The prohibitions were unavailing. Sports persisted and multiplied. By the end of the 14th Century, there were 1,400 professional tennis masters and untold numbers of amateurs in Paris alone. The authorities eventually gave in. In England, James I rescinded the British ban on games in the early 17th Century. He even gave soccer his particular blessing, pronouncing it an honorable pastime that built character and physical strength.

Today games still are the most popular form of exercise in the world. In Denmark, one person in four belongs to an athletic club. Sweden, a country of fewer than nine million people, has 35,000 amateur sports clubs. In the United States, some 25 million people participate each year in contests officially sanctioned by the Amateur Athletic Union (AAU), and untold millions, of both sexes and all ages, compete in games sponsored by municipal recreation leagues and such diverse organizations as the United States Tennis Association, the Amateur Hockey Association of the United

States and the United States Racquetball Association. Women's leagues have expanded and now include not just the traditional field hockey and volleyball but contact sports such as basketball, soccer and rugby as well.

It is not hard to see why so many people prefer to get their exercise by participating in sports. Unlike conventional exercise programs, which consist primarily of monotonous, solitary labor, games promise excitement and variety. They offer the personal pride to be gained by refining difficult skills: Tennis players strive to perfect a topspin backhand or a pinpoint serve, golfers master drives, chips and putts, virtuoso soccer players juggle the ball with their feet. And competition naturally fosters a camaraderie, both on the field and off, that has become an article of folklore throughout the world—the postgame revels of rugby players are reputedly as strenuous as the match itself.

Indeed, games have become so popular that exercises begun solely for their contribution to fitness are made into sports. Weekend races for runners, walkers, bicyclists, swimmers and cross-country skiers have become commonplace. Even such mammoth events as the New York Marathon are athletic contests only in a special sense. No more than about 100 entrants, world-renowned athletes, can hope for a chance to win the race; the 15,000 runners behind them are galvanized by their own competition, as they duel with other runners or with themselves, striving to better a previous time. They enjoy the company they find in what otherwise would be a solitary activity; the marathon is a protracted

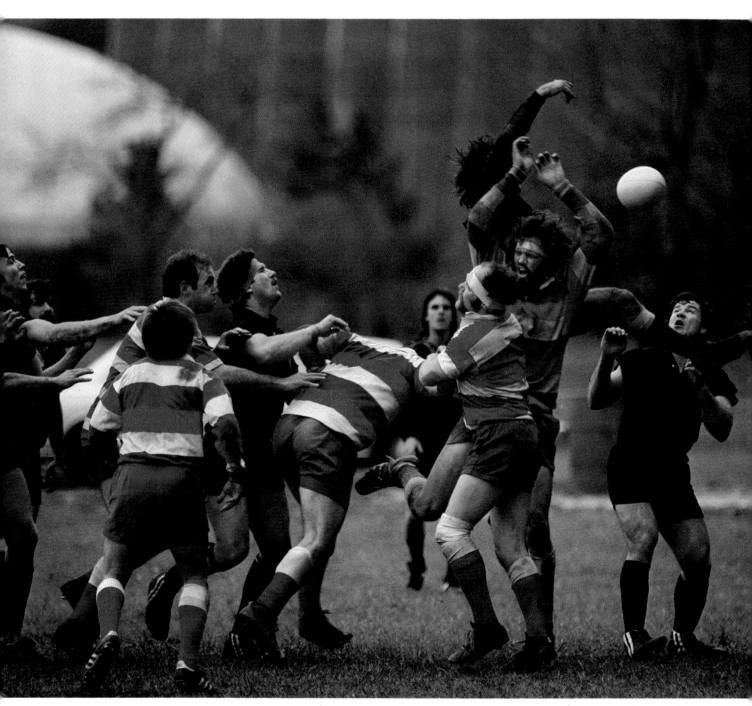

Amateur rugby teams from New York and Portland, Maine, clash over a melon-shaped leather ball in a contest that resembles American football. But with nonstop, 40-minute halves and no substitutions of players, rugby is a better sport for building overall physical fitness than the stop-and-start American game.

conversation, with ever-changing clusters of runners discussing training, fatigue and postrace parties. And of course all entrants look forward to popular acclaim. "The crowds are wonderful," said one. "They shout encouragement, hold out ice cubes on hot days, sprinkle you with water from hoses, offer soft drinks and peeled oranges."

Using sports as a means of exercising for fitness requires considerable perseverance, because health-promoting activities must be performed on a regularly repeated schedule, and practical obstacles invariably hinder anyone who tries to establish a settled routine of games three times a week or so. Outdoor sports generally are seasonal, and even during the season they are subject to the vagaries of the weather. Getting players together is complicated: A simple tennis match can be an administrative nightmare. Many sports also require special courts or fields whose use is difficult to schedule and often expensive as well.

Furthermore, because the health benefits of different sports vary widely—many are good fun but not very good exercise—games must be chosen carefully if they are expected to promote fitness. Stanford University's Dr. Ralph Paffenbarger, in his review of the health of 16,936 Harvard graduates of the classes of 1916 to 1950, discovered that the men who participated in popular but not very strenuous sports—bowling, baseball and golf, for example—suffered virtually the same number of heart attacks as those who did not exercise at all. The graduates who played games requiring more vigorous exertion, such as basketball, skiing and singles tennis, had only one third as many heart attacks as did the sedentary men.

With a few important exceptions, sports do not contribute much to the aerobic efficiency that improves the circulatory system, nor do they markedly increase strength and flexibility. They do not require sustained exertion sufficient to build endurance, they do not systematically overload muscles enough to build upper-body strength, and their movements do not stretch muscles and joints enough to improve flexibility. Yet all these characteristics are essential prerequisites to athletic ability. For this reason, anyone who takes up a sport, whether for physical conditioning or proficiency in the game,

must combine practice in sports technique with exercise routines. To supplement actual play, professional and amateur athletes alike are using modern research into sports to tailor exercise and practice programs to the particular demands of each sport and to get maximum health benefits. Such studies also have revised conventional thinking about the foods to be eaten before and during a game, and about treating an almost unavoidable concomitant of games: sports injuries.

Anyone who exercises regularly runs some risk of harm, of course, but the heat of competition dramatically increases the danger. Until recently sports injuries were treated primarily with rest. Today physiologists and physicians have discovered new ways to speed healing, often with simple home remedies. For serious cases, they have developed remarkable surgical procedures to repair injuries that would have proved crippling a few years ago.

The budding science of sports physiology

Unlike the standard exercises, games are difficult to examine scientifically. They demand complex, variable movements that defy laboratory analysis. The physiologist's unwieldy battery of instruments—treadmills, swimming flumes, bicycle ergometers, electrocardiographs and respirators—is useless on the playing field. Most portable instruments, such as the huge air bags used to measure the oxygen consumption of cross-country skiers, are too cumbersome for fast-moving competitive games. Some revealing experiments cannot even be approximated on the playing field; blood samples, for example, can be taken as an athlete runs on a treadmill, pedals a stationary bicycle or lifts weights, but not while a game is in progress.

Accordingly most research into the physiology of sports is done indirectly, by combining laboratory findings with on-the-field experiments. To determine the aerobic demands of a game, for example, scientists first test a player on a treadmill, charting his heart rate against the chemical content of the exhaled air to calculate oxygen consumption and energy consumption. They then wire the athlete with electrodes and a miniature transmitter that radios his heart rate during a game to a recorder on the sidelines. The heart rate in the field

Natalie Bacon, confined to a wheelchair, struggles uphill
in the 1979 running of the 7.5-mile Falmouth race on Cape Cod.
Wheelchair racers compete in special divisions of many
foot races. Their remarkable strength, when combined with the
speed advantage of rolling wheels, enables some of them
to finish ahead of the fastest runners.

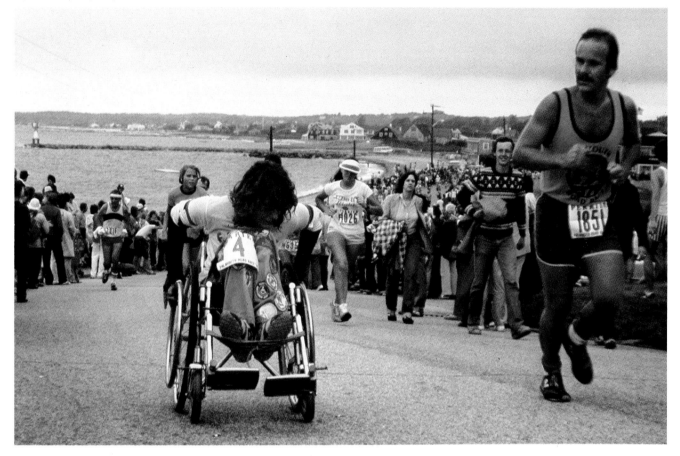

is matched against heart rates measured on the treadmill; this yields an estimate of oxygen consumption during the game.

Such extrapolations depend on the assumption that physical demands in the laboratory experiments are equivalent to those of a game—a reasonable belief, but one that physiologists readily admit they cannot prove. Games may introduce uncontrolled, unmeasurable variables that skew the experimental results. Complex movements during the game may make oxygen demands different from those of running on a treadmill—and heart rates can be driven up simply by the excitement of competition.

Despite these methodological weaknesses, the experiments have evaluated the benefits to be gained from sports

and have illuminated the scientific basis of sports performance, in the process confirming a few tenets of the folk wisdom that pervades sports and revising many others.

Which games are good for you

The most important findings of recent research into sports make it possible to rate the games for their value as exercise. Most games are surprisingly ineffective, and they are particularly unhelpful in improving the aerobic capacity that is considered essential for fitness. For aerobic benefit an activity should raise the heart rate into the target zone and keep it there for at least 20 minutes. During a game, a player's pulse rate never climbs predictably to a plateau, as it would during

Coaching athletes with a computer

During most of his javelin-throwing career, Olympic athlete Bill Schmidt had bent his left knee as he hurled the eight-foot lance. But after he was coached by a computer *(right)*, he began to keep his knee rigid. After one month with the new technique, he raised the average length of his throws by 20 feet.

The computer coach that helped Schmidt win an Olympic medal was developed by Gideon Ariel, holder of a doctorate in exercise science. Using a slow-motion movie of Schmidt in action, Ariel plotted the position of 16 joints every 1/100 second during the two seconds it takes to throw a javelin.

The 3,200 positions that resulted were fed into Ariel's computer, which measured how fast and far each of Schmidt's body segments moved, and from these data calculated the force Schmidt imparted to the javelin as he threw it. Then, on a stick figure of the action produced by the computer, Ariel repositioned Schmidt's joints slightly to see if a different throwing style would be more forceful. He calculated that Schmidt, by keeping his knee rigid and coordinating his movements perfectly, had the potential for a 300-foot throw.

In studying champions, Ariel has made discoveries that anyone can use to improve athletic performance and thus increase the value of many sports as exercise. His conclusions:
• You can put more punch into your tennis serve by keeping both feet on the ground, thus transmitting some of the strength in your legs through your arm.
• You can add spring to a basketball or volleyball jump if you bend your knee no more than halfway and thrust up with your arms.
• If you play hockey, you can speed up your slap shot by bending your stick against the ice just before it strikes the puck. The stick acts as a spring that rockets the puck toward the goal.

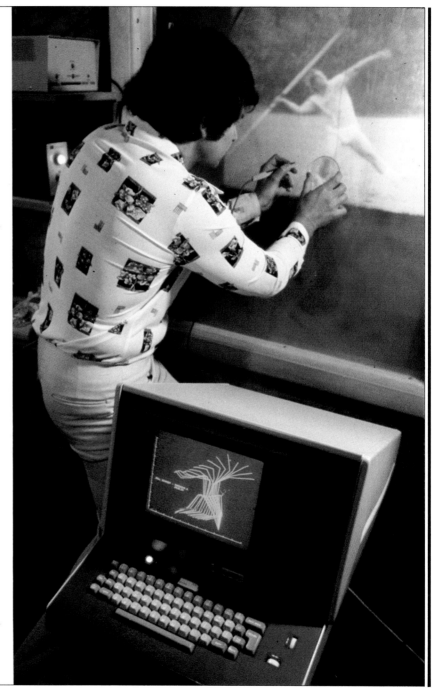

Touching a sonic stylus to a sound-sensitive movie screen, Gideon Ariel marks the location of Bill Schmidt's knee in a movie of Schmidt throwing a javelin. Tiny microphones along the edges of the screen pick up the sound of the stylus and flash the position of the athlete's knee to a computer that converts such data into a flowing stick figure, which it analyzes for flaws in movement.

some steady activity such as jogging or swimming. Instead it oscillates wildly. Charts of players' heart rates show a mountain range of peaks and valleys as the pulse rate pops in and out of the target zone. "Most types of ball games represent more or less intermittent work with frequent interchanges of short bursts of physical effort interspaced with brief pauses," wrote Swedish physiologists Drs. Per-Olof Åstrand and Kaare Rodahl. "For this reason, ball games have not required the same level of aerobic power as continuous, long-lasting effort of near-maximal intensity."

Even among champion athletes, aerobic capacity varies considerably with their sport. A study of Swedish athletes revealed that participants in short events, such as gymnastics, weight lifting and wrestling, had an average VO_2 max of about 53 milliliters, only slightly above the average score of 45 for nonathletic Swedes in the same age group. Players of soccer, basketball and ice hockey scored about 60 milliliters, along with fencers and ski jumpers. Badminton players scored 65 milliliters, just below the level of rowers and canoeists. By contrast, athletes from endurance sports—those that most resemble common exercises and are less popular as competitive games—had significantly higher average scores: Swimmers and walkers scored about 70 milliliters, speed skaters and bicyclists about 75 milliliters, middle-distance runners 80 milliliters, and long-distance runners and cross-country skiers about 85 milliliters. These measurements of athletes indicate which kinds of games can provide aerobic benefits.

The longer a game's performance time—the time actually consumed by physical activity—the greater its aerobic benefit. Performance time in this sense excludes all interruptions—time-outs, huddles, out-of-bounds plays, pauses between points and the like.

The more strenuous a sport, the better its aerobic benefit. Exertion depends not only on the demands of the sport, but also on the competition. In tennis, for example, Dr. Ralph Paffenbarger said, "Batting the ball around on Sunday with young children generally isn't strenuous, but a stiff, competitive game of singles is." Even in a relatively inactive sport such as table tennis, fierce competition can increase aerobic

effort: In one study, a champion Swedish player's heart rate remained above 180 beats per minute for an entire 27-minute match, with an average rate of 189. During another match, however, a losing player's heart rate peaked at 175 beats per minute and gradually dropped to less than 130. The demands of a game also depend to some extent on the player's own level of skill and conditioning. A beginning tennis player spends most of his time chasing loose balls, and his heart rate rarely enters the target zone; accomplished amateurs often sustain two- or three-minute rallies, and thus derive considerable aerobic benefit from the sport.

According to these rules of thumb, games fit into three general groups:

● Sports that require extremely short bursts of exertion and allow long pauses between bursts, such as softball, American football, cricket, bowling and golf, rely almost exclusively on energy mechanisms that operate anaerobically, independently of oxygen. These sports confer virtually no aerobic benefit. Edward Fox, a physiology professor at The Ohio State University, estimates that football and golf do not use aerobic energy at all. In baseball and ice hockey, Professor Fox says, the anaerobic systems produce 90 per cent of the energy required and the aerobic system only 10 per cent.

● Sports that require slightly longer bursts of energy and allow only brief pauses between them—such as volleyball, tennis, squash, racquetball, handball and badminton—help somewhat in developing aerobic fitness. The interludes between points—that is, between spells of active play—usually allow a player's heart rate to slip below the target zone momentarily, but since it quickly accelerates again, his average heart rate—a rough yardstick of aerobic benefit—is fairly high. Fox estimates that volleyball, tennis and fencing are about 80 per cent anaerobic and 20 per cent aerobic.

● Continuous sports, such as rugby, soccer, lacrosse, downhill skiing, field hockey and basketball, are among the best games for aerobic training. But even they are primarily anaerobic: Fox estimates that soccer, lacrosse and field hockey are only 30 per cent aerobic. As exercise, they fall far short of the activities ordinarily pursued for health benefits. A two-mile run is 80 per cent aerobic; jogging and cross-country skiing are almost entirely aerobic.

Such facts can help in the choice of a sport for its contribution to fitness. But sports are undertaken for enjoyment as well as for fitness. Those who enjoy a sport the most excel at it; they have the skill, stamina, strength and flexibility to play well. Developing those attributes requires physical conditioning—conditioning that cannot be obtained simply by playing the game. Thus professional and amateur athletes alike use the results of modern research into sports to help them improve their performance.

The key discoveries have explained why different sports require different types of conditioning. There are three types of fitness that, singly or in combination, determine athletic potential. One, of course, is aerobic fitness—the primary goal of most exercise programs. But in games, which generally depend less on prolonged endurance than on strenuous exertion separated by lengthy pauses, two other types of fitness are predominant. Both operate anaerobically.

Sports such as football, baseball and bowling, along with sprint races, require extremely short bursts of energy and rely

exclusively on an anaerobic mechanism called the speed system, which makes use of chemical energy already stored in the muscles. This system, the body's sole source of instant muscular power, can provide energy for a very short time— less than 10 seconds of all-out exertion, barely enough time to complete a 100-yard dash.

Training can increase the supply of instant energy by as much as 40 per cent. One technique, used to develop running speed among players in virtually every sport, consists of a series of sprints, between 40 and 100 yards long, with a two- or three-minute pause after each run. Another, employed to develop the throwing arm of a pitcher or quarterback, requires him to throw as hard as he can, over and over. By repeatedly depleting the instant energy in the muscles, such regimens gradually enlarge storage capacity. This increase in capacity has the effect of increasing both a runner's top speed and the length of time that he can sustain it, and of enabling a pitcher or quarterback to throw harder.

In games that do not have long pauses between the points, such as volleyball and the racket sports, the muscles soon

Wheels and tracks for skiing without snow

New kinds of equipment, designed for rolling on dry land instead of sliding over snow, let the skier triumph over his environment and pursue a traditional winter exercise the year round. Several types of skis, all fairly expensive, have been designed for use on pavement or grass to simulate the actions of cross-country or downhill skiing.

Summer skis for cross-country enthusiasts have wheels and provide outstanding endurance exercise. For downhill buffs, tractor-tread skis, used on grass, closely approximate the effect of skiing on snow. But staying upright on such skis requires advanced skill, and there is no cushion of snow to fall into.

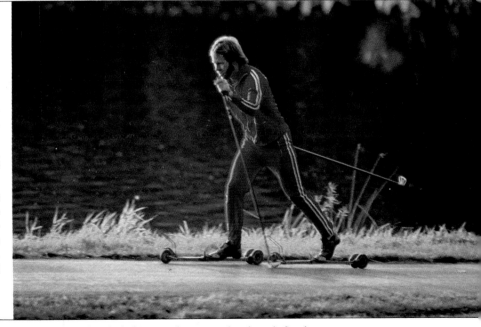

A summertime skier kicks his way along a road on boards fitted with wheels. A gear keeps the wheels from rolling backward and offers resistance simulating that of snow. The wires at the front brake the boards as they tilt during a fall.

begin to generate energy with a second anaerobic mechanism, by partially breaking down sugars stored in the muscles and, to a lesser extent, in the blood and elsewhere in the body. This mechanism, the intermediate process, provides only half the power of the speed system but lasts longer. Its duration is limited by the chemical by-products of the sugar breakdown, which accumulate to high levels after about two minutes of strenuous play, gradually sapping strength.

Recovery from such exercises is quite slow; in a resting athlete, half the chemical by-products are flushed away in 15 minutes, but the remainder are not completely purged for more than an hour. The speed of this recovery can be nearly doubled, however, by moderate exercise that is continued after strenuous exertion stops. Thus runners regain their strength at a faster rate by taking a victory lap after the end of a race, and players in football, soccer and similar games are best off loping back up the field after a long run, rather than stopping to recover their breath.

This intermediate system, which is the mainstay of most sports, also can be made more effective by training. Wind

sprints—20- to 100-yard sprints that are run 30 seconds to a minute apart—serve this purpose. A modern variation called interval training requires the athlete to run at a speed slightly below his maximum, jog easily until he partially recovers, and repeat this sequence several times, resting after every set of four or five runs; the distances and times vary according to the sport. These techniques repeatedly overload the intermediate energy system, building the muscles' ability to break down sugar and enhancing their tolerance for the intermediate system's chemical by-products.

The speed and intermediate systems, which operate independently of oxygen, are insufficient as energy sources for games that require steady, uninterrupted exertion, such as basketball, soccer and rugby. Anaerobic output declines after about two minutes and must be replaced by energy derived from reactions requiring oxygen. Such aerobic reactions provide an efficient energy-generating process that, unlike the anaerobic systems, uses plentiful fuel sources, produces no exercise-inhibiting chemical by-products and can continue for a long time—hours if necessary.

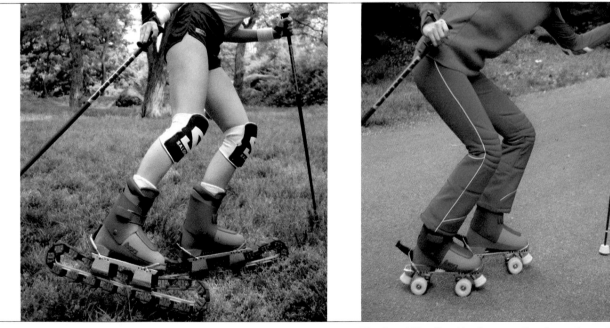

Tractor-tread grass skis turn any stretch of downhill turf into a ski run. Because they do not permit lateral slipping or cutting into turns as snow skis do, they demand considerable skill from the user and are most valuable to experienced skiers.

The downhill roller skis above—roller skates clamped to ski boots—are for use on pavement. They serve for practicing the twisting route of the slalom—summer skiers mark off the turns with beer cans on a sloping stretch of road.

The lag between the start of a game and the response of the aerobic system is the time needed for the heart and lungs to begin delivering the extra oxygen required for aerobic reactions. As the lungs take in more air, they begin exchanging oxygen and carbon dioxide efficiently, and heart rate and breathing rate increase. Only then, after three to five minutes, does the aerobic system become the primary source of muscular energy. Often this transition is palpable. Physiologists believe that "second wind," the subjective feeling that arises when labored breathing and crushing fatigue at the beginning of a contest give way to a smoother rhythm, reflects more efficient breathing and better blood circulation. And they theorize that the painful "stitch in the side" that sometimes afflicts athletes at the start of a game may be caused by poor blood circulation to chest muscles that are straining to increase air intake.

In addition to supplying energy directly to the muscles for steady exertion, the aerobic system has another essential role: It determines how promptly the anaerobic speed and intermediate systems can recover after exhaustion and again provide their quick action. This consideration is unimportant to athletes who rely on a single burst of energy followed by a long pause, such as sprinters and outfielders. But it is essential in continuous games, such as basketball and soccer; and in intermittent ones that allow only brief pauses between points, such as volleyball and the racket sports. An aerobically conditioned athlete is better able than an untrained one to maintain his responses at their initial level—and this is an advantage that often proves decisive, particularly toward the end of a match.

This crucial relationship between the aerobic and anaerobic systems was dramatically illustrated in 1973 when Bobby Riggs, a 55-year-old former men's tennis champion of limited endurance, challenged 29-year-old Billie Jean King, a superbly conditioned women's champion. Riggs, vowing to prove that male players were naturally superior to women regardless of their ages, held his own briefly at the start of the match, breaking King's serve in the first set—but she immediately rallied to break him in the next game. King continued to play steadily and went on to defeat her exhausted opponent

in three straight sets. "He didn't have time to recover between points," observed a physiologist who watched the match. "He progressively suffered from fatigue and it eventually affected his skill."

The importance of aerobic capacity to athletic prowess in many sports is now widely recognized, and athletes build their capacity the same way other people do, by running. They also pay close attention to other factors that affect performance—food, smoking, atmospheric conditions—and they make use of special calisthenics that provide muscles and joints with the degree of strength and flexibility needed to play well and avoid injury.

Eating to play better

Speed, strength and endurance—three key components of success in virtually any sport—are determined in large part by the amount of energy available to the athlete's muscles. This in turn is determined by the availability of oxygen and other raw materials to power the muscles and flush away chemical wastes. Coaches long have recognized the connection between food, air and sports performance—and have prescribed fad diets, training-table meals, oxygen inhalations and other gimmicks. Now physiologists have developed scientific evidence that proper diet and breathing habits can boost sports performance.

Athletes traditionally have eaten a high-protein diet, with plenty of red meat and milk—perhaps on the assumption that, since muscle fiber is made of protein, it needs to have protein for nourishment. Modern research has discredited that idea. Although muscles do need some protein food, the amount that is supplied by a balanced diet is more than sufficient for any athlete.

Now it is known that an athlete's diet should contain a high proportion not of proteins but of carbohydrates, such as are found in bread, potatoes, pasta, cereal and vegetables. Carbohydrates make up the raw material that provides much of the body's muscular power, they are easy to digest and they readily break down into glucose, the simple sugar on which the muscles' biochemical processes depend for most of their energy. A high-carbohydrate diet allows the muscles

Strenuous pastimes from times past

Many sports are known and enjoyed the world over. Others are as unique to locality or ethnic tradition as the caber toss *(right)* of Scotland, the log birling of the North American forests, or Dutch canal vaulting *(pages 124-125)*.

Tossing the caber, or tree trunk, is typical of these oldtime sports in its celebration of strength combined with an esoteric skill. The caber is a tapered wooden pole, roughly 16 to 18 feet long and weighing about 100 pounds (the exact dimensions have never been standardized, a vagueness that is part of the charm of such sports).

Little known outside Scottish communities, caber tossing is still the climactic event of the Highland Games performed each summer in dozens of Scotland's villages and in other parts of the world settled by Scots. To the music of bagpipe bands, burly Scotsmen take their turns in the event. Each man lifts the caber as best he can, clasping his hands beneath the narrow end and bracing the pole against a shoulder. Then, after a few lurching steps, he flings the caber forward.

The winner is not necessarily the man who tosses the caber farthest. More important, and more heavily weighted in the judging, is the trajectory of a toss: The pole should trace a high arc and drop forward, pointing straight away from the man who tossed it.

His face contorted with effort, a competitor in the Highland Games near Edinburgh, Scotland, heaves a caber into the air. The toss calls for skill as well as brute strength, and takes years of practice; many champions are in their fifties.

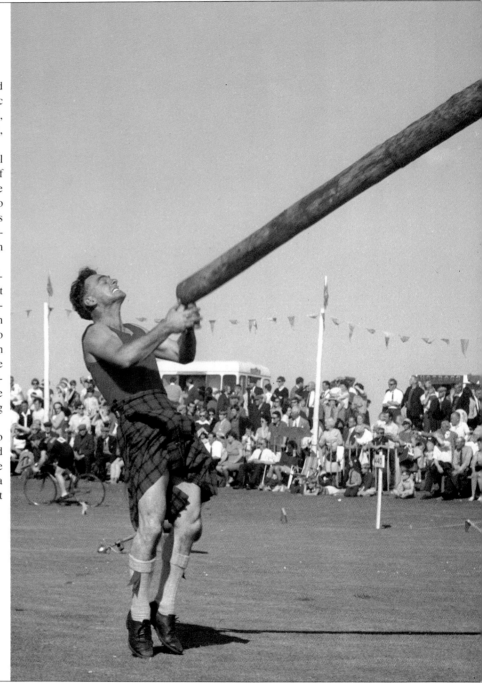

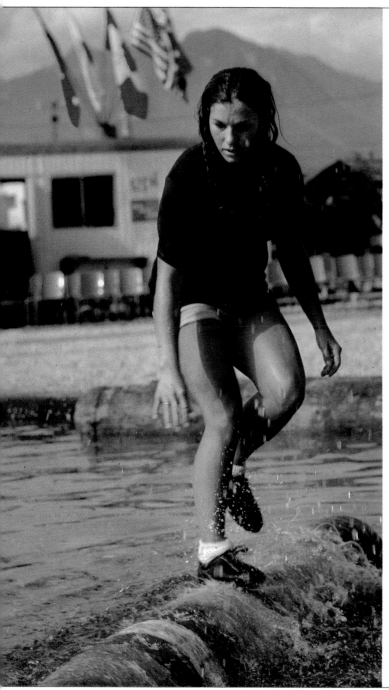

At a timber carnival in British Columbia, Canada, a young woman spins a slippery log in the now-liberated but once purely male sport of birling, originated by North American lumberjacks. In competitive birling two opponents share a log, abruptly changing its spin as they attempt to fling each other into the icy water.

A contestant hurls a 185-pound stone in a folk sport called Unspunnen, popular among Swiss farmers and herdsmen since the 14th Century. A national contest is held at La Chaux-de-Fonds every three years; the 1980 winner set a record of 3.7 yards, and won the traditional award: a cowbell.

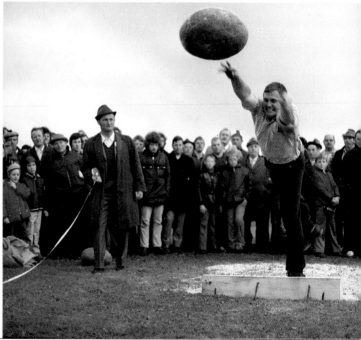

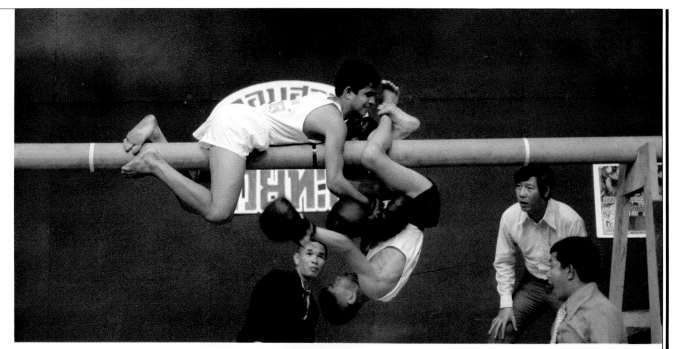

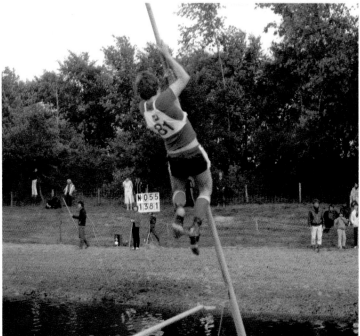

Clinging precariously to a wooden bar, Thai sea boxers pummel each other in a tournament version of an ancient sport; the match will end when one fighter tumbles to a cushioned mat below. As originally practiced, sea boxing was literally that: Thai sailors fought astride a ship's boom that extended high over the water.

A ljepper flies across a canal in Holland. Unlike an ordinary pole vaulter, the ljepper tries for distance, not height. He sprints to the canal bank, leaps to a pole resting on a yellow cradle (bottom), then shinnies up it as it rises with the force of his leap. Finally, he releases the pole and lands on the far side of the canal.

to store about .6 ounce of glycogen—a form of glucose—per pound of body weight, nearly twice as much as a normal diet would supply.

One experiment compared normal and high-carbohydrate diets by testing 10 distance runners in two 30-kilometer (19-mile) races. Three weeks before the first race, six of the runners began a high-carbohydrate diet while the other four continued with a normal diet; after the race the groups switched diets for three weeks, then raced again. While on the carbohydrate diet, both groups of subjects ran an average of eight minutes faster than they could on the normal diet.

Some athletes carry the high-carbohydrate regimen to an extreme, using a procedure called carbohydrate loading to concentrate glycogen in their bodies. About a week before competition, they exercise until exhausted, depleting the glycogen supply almost completely. For the next three days they train moderately and live mainly on fats and proteins, eating virtually no carbohydrates—a diet that leaves them faint and dizzy. Then, three days before competition, they switch to a high-carbohydrate diet and simultaneously reduce their training to conserve muscle energy. This radical technique, used only under a physician's supervision, can increase the glycogen stored in the body and available for conversion into energy by more than 300 per cent.

The meal just before a game is critical for athletes. Physiologists recommend that a high-carbohydrate meal be eaten at least three hours before competition, to allow time for complete digestion. If less time is available, a smaller meal is prescribed—cereal and milk, for example—at least 30 minutes before the game. Athletes generally avoid hard-to-digest foods that might make them feel full and sluggish—those that are high in proteins or fats, or are oily, highly spiced or

How sports score as exercise

Exercise to play a good game; do not play games to exercise. The validity of that advice is indicated by the graph below, which compares four common exercises with seven popular sports for their aerobic value in developing endurance. Based on Dr. Kenneth Cooper's determinations of oxygen consumption in the laboratory and on the playing field, the graph presents his findings in the point system he devised. The points listed are produced by 20 minutes' participation—30 points per week are considered necessary for aerobic improvement. The results are strikingly similar to comparisons of exercises for their effectiveness in the elimination of fat (page 47).

Running, swimming and cycling, which demand continuous, vigorous exertion, are best for aerobic fitness. Walking is as effective as basketball and soccer because it involves steady activity. And such sports as golf and doubles tennis, which involve more standing than movement, are almost useless.

Exercise / Sport	Aerobic value in points
Running (6 miles per hour)	
Swimming (40 yards per minute)	
Bicycling (15 miles per hour)	
Basketball	
Soccer	
Walking (4 miles per hour)	
Football	
Tennis (singles)	
Volleyball	
Golf (walking and carrying clubs)	
Tennis (doubles)	

AEROBIC VALUE IN POINTS (scale 0 to 8)

fibrous. They also avoid gas-producing foods such as onions, beans and cabbage.

For many years, athletes ate sweets—honey, candy, pastry and cakes—just before competition, on the theory that the sugar in such foods could increase the supply of the sugar compound that their muscles needed for energy. Recent experiments have proved just the opposite. High dosages of sweets impair athletic performance, because the extra glucose from their sugar has a backlash. If more sugar is consumed than the body can handle, the body automatically secretes chemicals that rapidly break down the excess. But then it overreacts. The chemical breakdown continues and the level of glucose in the blood is reduced to below normal. In the 1980 Winter Olympics, United States figure skater Linda Fratianne consumed several spoonfuls of honey just before she went onto the ice during the last competition, hoping to gain extra energy. She later said that she felt tired and listless instead—an effect physiologists attribute to an overdose of sugar.

Low dosages of glucose can provide some benefit. But even they have many limitations. Glucose becomes available for muscular energy only slowly, first taking hold at least 20 minutes after ingestion and having its greatest effect one to two hours later. In addition it retards the body's absorption of liquid from the stomach. In one Swedish experiment, young men drank several glucose solutions and then ran on a treadmill while the liquids in their stomachs were monitored. The results were striking. Cold solutions were absorbed much faster than warm ones, and dilute glucose solutions were absorbed faster than concentrated ones. In fact, concentrated solutions so retarded the passage of liquid out of the stomach that they could cause dehydration in a sweating athlete, regardless of how much water he drank, by preventing the water from leaving the stomach.

As a result of this research, physiologists now recommend glucose only for athletes engaged in events of moderate intensity lasting longer than two hours—a five-set tennis match, for example. To facilitate its absorption from the stomach, the solution should be cold and the glucose concentration should be no more than 2.5 per cent. Most endurance athletes mix unsweetened fruit juices or prepared drinks such as Gatorade half and half with water to get the right glucose concentration, and consume three to seven fluid ounces every 15 minutes during competition.

The muscles' ability to burn glucose and similar fuels depends to a great extent on aerobic fitness. But VO2max can be affected by the quality of the air a person breathes. Several experiments have demonstrated that air pollution at the levels encountered in many urban areas has negative effects on athletic performance, reducing aerobic capacity by about 10 per cent. In a study conducted at the University of California, six volunteers ran on a treadmill while breathing air containing ozone, a component of the smog that is commonly found in urban areas. After one hour all had impaired breathing. Their respiratory rates increased 25 per cent while their lung capacity decreased 30 per cent. Two of the subjects were so sensitive to ozone that they were not able to complete one hour of exercise at 65 per cent of their normal VO2max, a task they ordinarily could have done with ease.

On the basis of such studies, physiologists recommend that athletes avoid outdoor sports on smoggy days or, failing that, that they schedule practices and games in the morning, after rush hour, when pollutant levels are lower.

The most hazardous pollutant, of course, is cigarette smoke. Its damaging effect on aerobic capacity is more pronounced than that of ozone. If an athlete smokes a pack and a half a day, the carbon monoxide that he inhales in the tobacco smoke attaches itself to nearly 10 per cent of his blood's hemoglobin, which otherwise would be carrying oxygen to his muscles; this effect lingers for at least a day after the latest cigarette.

An influence of somewhat shorter duration was found in an experiment at the University of Toronto. Researchers there administered two treadmill tests to a group of regular smokers. One test was made after the smokers had abstained for a day, a second immediately after they resumed smoking. Smoking just before the test was found to increase frictional resistance in the lung passages by 30 per cent—enough to rob the muscles of 5 per cent of their potential oxygen supply. Concluded Edward Fox, "Athletes who cannot or will not 'kick the habit' may aid their performance by not smoking on the day of competition.''

Not only the quality but also the density of air available affects performance. Athletes who live near sea level and occasionally compete in high-altitude sports such as downhill skiing must cope with a decreased oxygen supply. The lower air pressure at high altitude—it decreases by 30 per cent at 10,000 feet—means that less oxygen enters the lungs, the lungs work less efficiently and, as a result, less oxygen reaches the muscles. Although breathing and heart rates all automatically increase to compensate, aerobic capacity decreases substantially.

In one experiment, 12 runners were divided into two groups, one training near sea level in Davis, California, the other at the United States Air Force Academy in Colorado Springs, at an elevation of 7,546 feet. After three weeks the groups switched training sites, then continued the experiment for another three weeks. The results for both groups were strikingly consistent. The average VO_2max on the first day at Colorado Springs was 17.4 per cent below the VO_2max the same runners had at sea level, and the initial time for a two-mile run was 7.2 per cent longer. Even after three weeks of high-altitude training, the runners' average VO_2max was 14.8 per cent below that at sea level and the average two-mile time was 5.2 per cent longer.

Over a period of months at high altitude, the lungs become more efficient and the body manufactures extra hemoglobin, so that the blood can transport more oxygen. This process eases the subjective feelings of strain at high altitude, but it never wholly compensates. Even athletes who live all year round in the mountains have less aerobic power at home than they do at sea level.

To allow for these effects, most athletes who travel to high-altitude competitions try to arrive at least a day or two before beginning strenuous exertion so that the respiratory and circulatory systems can begin their adjustments. Training intensity usually is reduced, because the aerobic system is quickly exhausted at high altitude. And because recovery from exhaustion takes much longer at high altitude than at sea level, athletes generally pace themselves carefully.

Air and food are simply the raw materials that the lungs and circulatory system help deliver to the muscles for conversion into energy. How effectively that energy is used depends on the strength and flexibility of the muscles and joints. All sports require strength, but not to the same extent; and flexibility, while valuable, can paradoxically be a hazard, leading to injury. Each attribute can be adjusted to the specific needs of a sport by special training techniques.

Building strength for athletics

According to a Greek legend, Milo of Crotona, seeking to become the strongest man in the world, began lifting a young bull calf to his shoulders when he was a boy. By the time the boy and his bull were fully grown, this regimen had helped make Milo the champion wrestler of the Sixth Century B.C.

The basic principles of building strength by steadily and repeatedly overloading the muscles have not changed much since Milo's day. Barbells and weight machines have superseded bulls, but weight training still is the main strength-building method for sports, and it is used by players of virtually every game.

Recent research, however, has revealed subtleties that have revised the application of weight training to sports conditioning. According to current theories, strength is a product not only of bigger, stronger muscles but of more efficient activation of muscles by the nervous system. This neural component of strength apparently is learned by the body. An Ohio State University study comparing high school and college swimmers found that, even when their form and physical conditioning were identical, the performance of the university athletes was far superior. This is an indication, said physiologists Donald Mathews and Edward Fox, that the college athletes ''were more skillful neuromuscularly and hence used their energy stores more efficiently.''

Neuromuscular skill depends both on the muscle that is being used and on the movement. The arm curl, for example—in which a dumbbell is held with the arm straight down, and the elbow is flexed until the dumbbell touches the shoulder—builds the biceps, the muscle of the upper arm. But this exercise does not provide much added strength for

The pros' arabesques and leapfrog

In the months when he does not play basketball for the Houston Rockets, guard Calvin Murphy stays in shape by twirling a baton—and has become so accomplished that he leads classes in it. Murphy bicycles and skips rope, too, but he swears by twirling as an exercise for the upper body: ''It makes me use the muscles in my chest and arms,'' he says.

More and more, professional athletes and their coaches are seeking unusual forms of exercise. The Washington, D.C., Diplomats soccer team begins practice workouts with a session of ''keep away,'' a children's game in which players arranged in a circle toss a ball among themselves while a man in the middle tries to intercept it. The drill is a useful warm-up, and it appeals to men who play games for a living. ''They may be professional athletes,'' says Diplomats trainer Steve Hornor, ''but they're still kids at heart.''

On the practice field, rapid-fire calisthenics are giving way to slow, limb-stretching exercises inspired by such unlikely disciplines as yoga and the dance. Gradual flexing, many trainers believe, stretches muscles better, making them more resistant to injury. And athletes will try anything—including an arabesque—to stay off the disabled list.

With the grace of a ballet dancer, the great power hitter Reggie Jackson of the New York Yankees executes a stretching exercise. During training in Fort Lauderdale, Florida, Jackson regularly combines 15 of these stretches, designed to extend the hamstring muscles, with weight lifting and sprints.

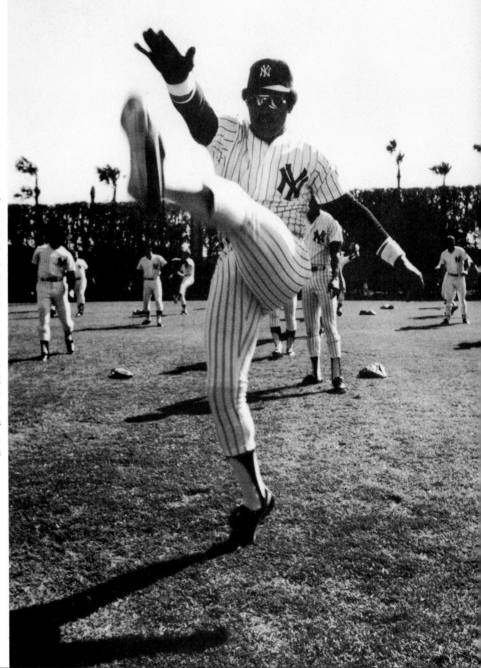

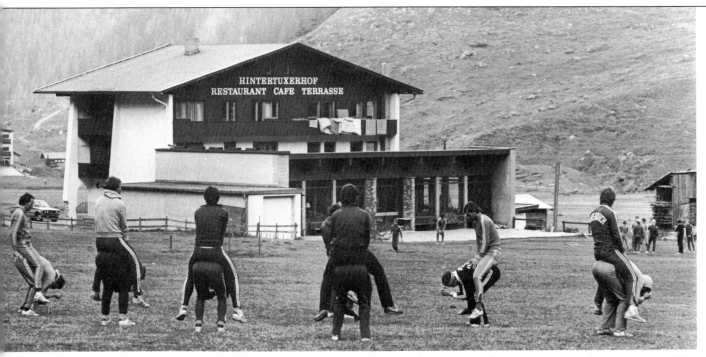

In an awkward game of horse and rider, men of the Austrian National Ski Team train for winter tournaments near Innsbruck. In each pair of men, the one at the bottom assumes the semicrouch of downhill skiing, then bounces forward while his partner straddles him. The exercise builds the quadriceps, the front thigh muscles that raise or lower a skier's body.

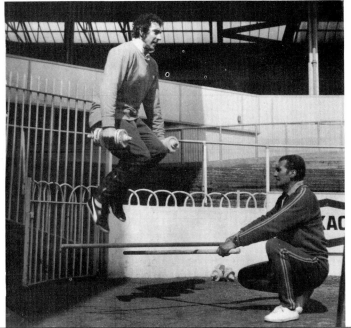

A coach wields a pair of broom handles as if they were the swords of a saber dance, to sharpen the reflexes of British soccer star Martin Chivers, who leaps up and out of the way— holding dumbbells—whenever the sticks come near him. Over the 40 repetitions in each session, the coach accelerates the pace to make Chivers' heart and lungs work harder.

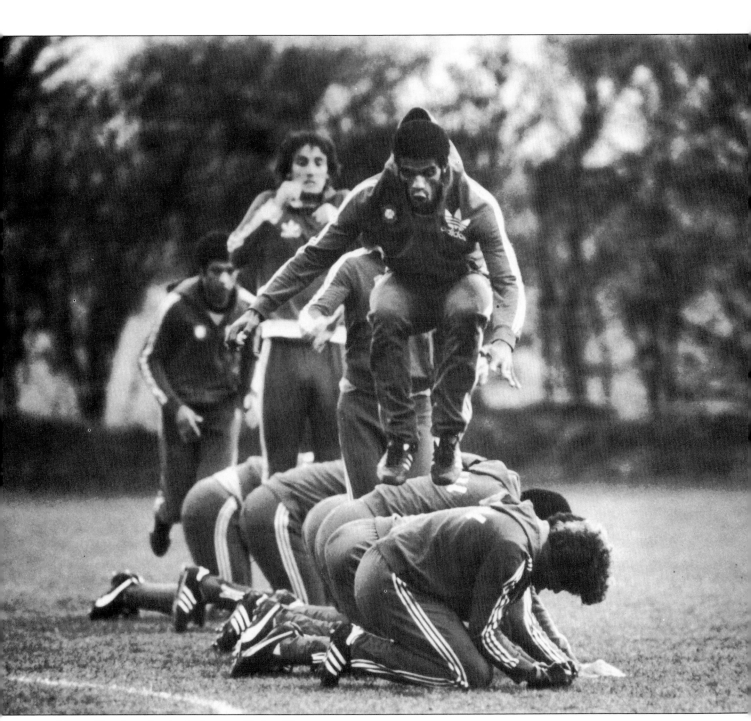

*A form of leapfrog absorbs the Brazilian National Soccer
Team. After each player hurdles his teammates, he kneels at the
end of the line; at the same moment, the man at the other
end of the line springs up to keep the routine going. This warm-up
exercise is especially useful for soccer players, who may
run six miles in the course of a game.*

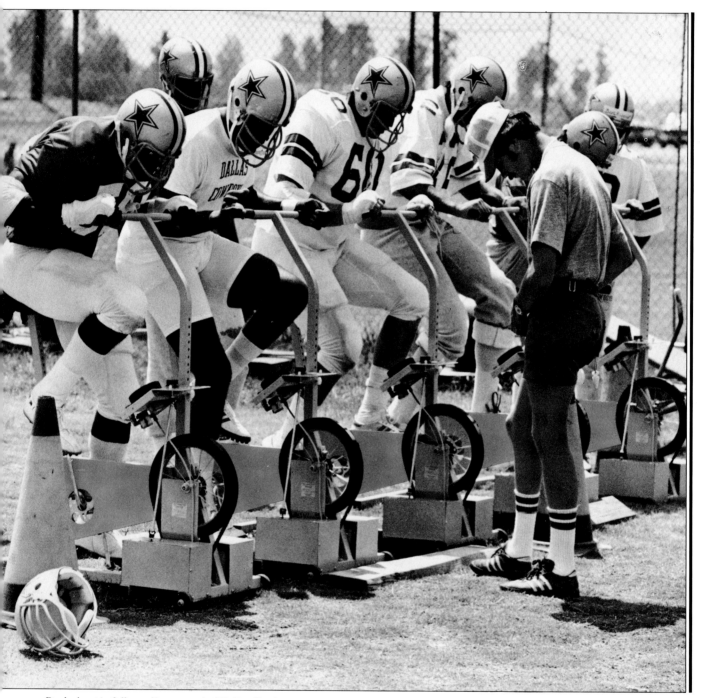

Decked out in full regalia, a squad of Dallas Cowboys labors on exercise bicycles. Cycling has long been practiced as an aerobic exercise, but these Cowboys are using specially rigged machines to mend injuries to knee and leg muscles. When a player pushes the pedals at a predetermined speed, the bike automatically "pushes back" with equal force.

lifting a weight up off the floor, or for a tennis stroke or a golf swing. If weight training is to improve strength for a sport, the movement of the weight should duplicate the movements of that particular sport.

Football linemen concentrate on pushing weights away in the bench press, while quarterbacks and baseball pitchers practice pull-overs that mimic the motion of throwing a ball. In addition to imitating the general course of a movement, effective weight training must also duplicate the speed and the angle of maximum exertion. The usual exercises with weights are performed slowly. Only a small portion of the strength gained in this way can be applied to the lightning movements needed for sports. Furthermore, the actual load on the muscles varies considerably at different points in a given exercise. In an arm curl, for example, it is relatively difficult to raise the dumbbell from the starting position; when the arm is straight, the muscle is strained almost to its limit. But lifting the weight becomes easy as the forearm passes the horizontal. As a result, at every angle other than the initial one—including many angles used in sports—the exercise builds relatively little strength.

To match all aspects of a weight-training motion—direction, speed and angle—to those of a sport, engineers and physiologists have developed so-called isokinetic machines, which are too expensive and bulky for home use but are available in some health clubs. The speed of an exercise is controlled hydraulically or by the friction of springs or chains. The machines can be set for fast speeds, developing the quickness needed for sports, and they stress muscles to their maximum throughout the full range of motion if the athlete continuously applies full force.

The isokinetic machines build strength much more quickly than barbells can—even when strength is measured by the subject's proficiency with barbells. In a study at the University of California at Davis, eight weeks of machine training produced 4 per cent greater strength gains than barbell exercises; in high-speed machine tests, machine training nearly doubled strength while barbell training had virtually no effect. The ultimate test was a series of events that approximated the demands of games—the broad jump, 40-yard dash,

softball throw, vertical jump and two-handed shot-put. In these events, men who trained on machines improved by about 5 per cent overall; men who trained with barbells showed no significant improvement.

Despite their impressive results in laboratory tests, even isokinetic exercises cannot exactly reproduce motions required by a game. For this reason, athletes in sports that require speed and skill more than raw power, such as tennis and soccer, rely less on barbells and machines than on practicing the actions of their particular game in some way that puts extra load on the muscles.

Tennis players leave the covers on their rackets to increase air resistance to the swing, then go through each stroke—forehand, backhand and serve—about 50 times; eventually they stuff tennis balls under the cover to add weight and to stress their muscles still more. Soccer and basketball players occasionally practice passing with a medicine ball, which weighs at least twice as much as an ordinary ball. Such training always is done in moderate doses and artificial situations. The medicine ball is used to build arm and chest muscles, not to improve technique. If athletes actually played with extra-heavy equipment, even in practice—if a tennis player tried to hit balls with an overweight racket or a pitcher threw a heavier ball—their timing and coordination with normal equipment would be thrown off.

Flexibility: too tight or too loose?

In addition to strength, games frequently require the muscles to deliver its exact opposite: supple, unresisting flexibility. A powerful tennis serve, for example, depends on flexibility in the shoulder and elbow. In the moment before the serve, a player's muscles must be loose enough to allow his arm and racket to coil far behind his back, so that the forward swing builds speed over the longest possible arc. Similar flexibility is required in baseball—for an overhand pitch, the pitcher's forearm rotates back until it is horizontal, a feat that few laymen can accomplish. Flexibility is important for another reason as well: Limber muscles generally absorb the shock of quick movements without injury, while tight ones all too often tear or "pull" at a critical moment.

Basketball: a game invented for fitness

Most team sports do little to promote fitness. Basketball is an exception. In a full-court game a player burns calories and builds aerobic capacity at a rate exceeded only by such pure exercises as swimming and running. The fact is not surprising: Dr. James Naismith, who invented the game in 1891, had "health-giving exercise" in mind.

An instructor and coach at a Massachusetts school for YMCA officials, Naismith was assigned to find an indoor sport to occupy the students during the winter. In response, he formulated what he called a "neat and nimble" game; his students approved, and introduced basketball to their hometown YMCAs.

In just one year, leagues were formed to schedule games for dozens of Ys, and the sport quickly became a fixture in YMCAs and schools around the world. "I merely hoped that it would persist a few years," wrote Naismith with wonderment. "I had no idea that it would gain so in popularity."

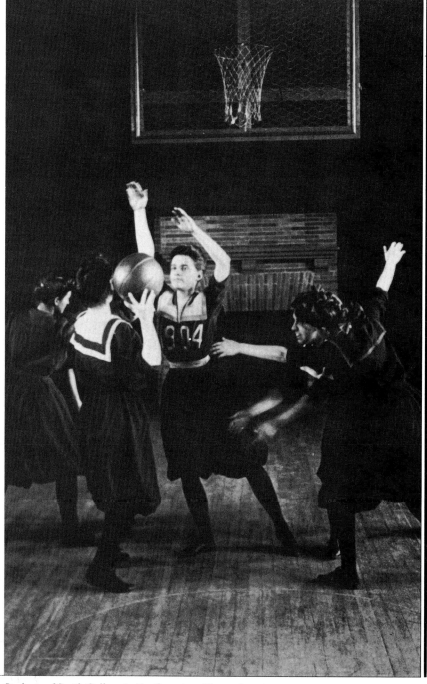

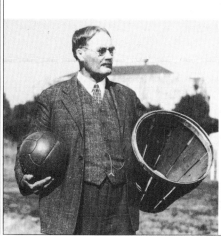

The game's paraphernalia are displayed by its inventor, Dr. James Naismith. Peach baskets were goals for the first contest because Naismith could not find what he really wanted—square wooden boxes.

Students of Smith College in Northampton, Massachusetts, take to the court in a converted gym, where the net hangs over a fireplace. Basketball, introduced at Smith in 1892, quickly became a favorite at American women's colleges; by 1930 more than 95 per cent of them provided facilities for the sport.

On the other hand, extreme flexibility can be a serious problem. If the muscles surrounding a joint are unusually pliable, whether from previous injury, an overzealous stretching program or an athlete's genetic make-up, they no longer adequately reinforce the joint. As the joint is forced to its normal limits—when an athlete plants his foot awkwardly, falls out of control or runs into another player—it must absorb the entire force. It sometimes gives way, resulting in a sprain or, in severe cases, a dislocation. This can happen to any joint, but in sports it occurs most often in the ankle and knee. Since flexibility, like strength, varies with each muscle and movement, a player may have one or two leg joints that sprain easily—a trick knee, for example—even if his other joints are not abnormally flexible.

Not surprisingly, the solutions to these two problems are diametrically opposed. To reinforce joints that are very loose, the surrounding muscles must be built up by exercises prescribed by an orthopedic surgeon. Overly tight muscles can be relaxed by stretching exercises such as those on pages 92-97, but some exercises are particularly good for some sports. Tennis players, for example, are especially susceptible to groin pulls, so they concentrate on groin exercises such as the one on page 94. Soccer players, prone to ankle injuries, often stretch this critical joint by walking for about 25 yards on the outside edges of their feet. Basketball and volleyball players are subject to back injuries; they do flattened and rounded back stretches, page 95.

Following such drills, players begin a warm-up of relaxed practice, gradually building to full intensity, because a sudden switch from static stretching to all-out play would risk injury. In addition, a warm-up helps by literally warming the muscles about 3° F. and raising the body's central temperature about 2° F. Laboratory tests have shown that elevated temperature improves several key elements of athletic performance: Flexibility increases about 20 per cent; blood vessels dilate, reducing the frictional resistance of the cardiovascular system 13 per cent; hemoglobin in the blood transports oxygen more efficiently, increasing VO_2max 8 per cent; and chemical reactions in the muscles speed up, making the muscle as much as 10 per cent stronger and faster. The combined effect of warmth is considerable. In one experiment, warm-ups increased the distance of a softball throw about seven feet.

Athletes today are acutely conscious of the importance of warmth. Even in well-heated gymnasiums, basketball players now leave their sweatsuits on during much of the pregame warm-up, to make sure that their body temperature rises. And several professional football teams, recognizing that players suffer more sprains and muscle pulls during cold weather, provide benches that blast warm air through vents onto players' legs and backs.

Treating injuries

Despite these precautions, sports injuries are frighteningly prevalent. In the United States, about 20 million weekend athletes and another 10 million school children are hurt each year. Most injuries do not require medical attention. Among those that do need treatment, the most common fall into three general categories.

• Muscle strains or "pulls" are characterized by searing pain in a muscle during strenuous exertion; the pain soon subsides to a dull ache. These strains are caused by an actual tear through part or all of a muscle. The area around the injury generally swells and discolors, like a bruise; the muscle itself may go into spasm. A slight tear may heal in a week, but a severe one requires three weeks for new muscle fibers to knit together and two or three months for the fibers to regain their original size and strength. Athletes sometimes mistakenly equate muscle pulls and tendon pulls. Tendons, the cords that anchor muscle to bone, are stronger than muscles, so they seldom rupture. When they do, they break with an audible, excruciating snap. Such injuries require immediate medical attention.

• Joint sprains, most commonly of the ankle or knee, are caused by a partial or complete rupture of a ligament—one of the cords that connect bone to bone, holding each joint together. They occur when a joint is forced beyond its normal range of motion. Sprains are accompanied by sharp pain whenever the joint is moved, and they generally swell quickly. The severity of the injury depends on the extent of liga-

Three common pains and how to avoid them

Some of the pains that plague active people show up in unexpected places. A basketball game, for example, may leave shins aching as though an opponent had been hurling the ball at them. Or an elbow throbs after a tennis match, although it was the muscles in the forearm and legs that were exerted.

Three common injuries of this type are diagramed at right. They are seldom the result of a blow or a single instance of overexertion. Rather, they build up slowly, from stresses caused by small misalignments in the swing of a racket or the position of a running foot. The stresses travel along the muscles, weakening the tendons, which connect muscles and bones, or puling one bone out of position so that it rubs painfully against another.

These ailments are not serious, but they get worse if ignored. The immediate remedy is rest, to give the damaged tissue time to repair itself; an ice pack on the painful area may relieve swelling and tenderness. Then, when the joint or muscle returns to normal, reinjury can be prevented by changing technique.

Tennis elbow can be avoided by using the backhand technique at near right. A two-handed backhand also may prevent injury.

Knee or leg injuries originating in the foot are trickier. A frequent source of the problem is overpronation—the result of a stride in which the foot hits the ground and rolls too far toward its inner side, flattening the arch and tugging at adjacent muscles. Overpronation is normal for many runners. But running on softer surfaces, such as grass, cushions the impact on leg muscles. Good running shoes (pages 76-77) also absorb shock and hold the heels firmly, minimizing the foot's tendency to waver. Orthopedic devices for the feet also may help; foam-rubber supports to boost sagging arches are sold at drugstores.

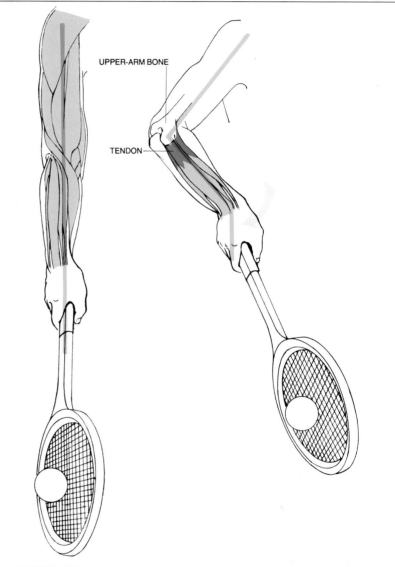

UPPER-ARM BONE

TENDON

TENNIS ELBOW
In a correct backhand stroke (left), the arm and racket form a nearly straight line when the ball is hit; the muscles (pink) of the upper arm and forearm absorb the impact. If the player crooks the elbow and snaps the wrist (right), forearm muscles alone take the impact and deliver it to a tendon linking them to the upper-arm bone. Such stress on the tendon causes elbow pain (red).

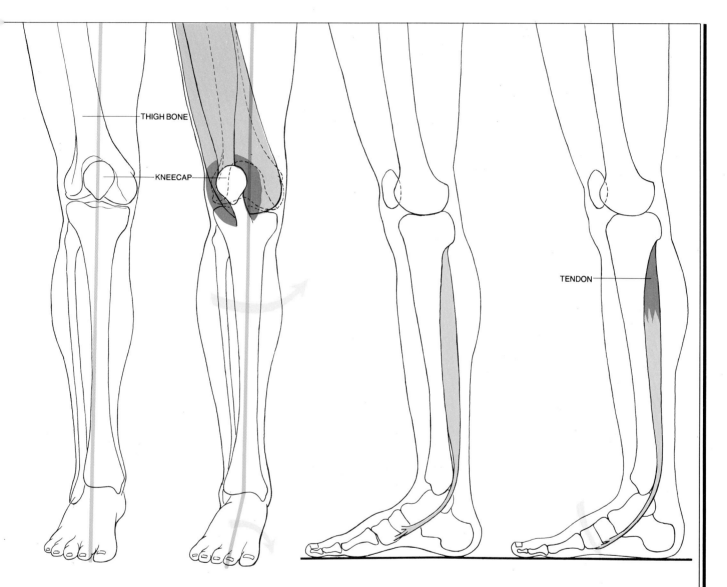

RUNNER'S KNEE

When a foot lands squarely during a run (left), the kneecap moves smoothly in a pocket between two ridges of the thigh bone. If the foot tilts in (right), so do the bones and muscles of the lower leg (arrows). To compensate, thigh muscles (pink) stretch outward, pulling the kneecap until it grinds against its bony pocket in the thigh bone (dashed lines), causing pain at the knee (red).

SHIN SPLINTS

Some of the muscles (pink) that let the foot tilt inward curve up into the calf (left). When a running foot tilts in (right, arrow) too far or too long, repeated pulls cause small tears in the tendon that anchors the muscle to the large leg bone and pain is felt in the calf and shin (red). As many as two thirds of all runners tilt their feet, risking the leg and knee problems shown on this page.

ment damage, which can range from the rupture of a few fibers to a complete break in the ligament. Since ligaments heal as slowly as bones, recovery from serious sprains may require six to 10 weeks. The joint may not become completely stable and pain-free for as long as four months.

● Overuse injuries—including swimmer's shoulder, runner's knee, tendinitis, shin splints and bursitis—are characterized by chronic, gradually building pain rather than sudden trauma. They are caused by simple wear and tear that irritates joints and tendons.

From Roman times until a few years ago, any of these injuries would have been treated with heat—hot baths, hot-water bottles or electric heating pads—on the assumption that, since heat speeds up metabolism generally, it also would speed the healing process. Modern research has proved just the opposite. Heat does speed up the bodily processes, but in doing so it stimulates injured tissue and dilates blood vessels; these reactions increase swelling and enlarge the pools of blood and fluid, slowing the healing process. Even in the absence of injury, heat following exercise can cause aches and pains. The ritual of a long, hot soak after a game creates pools of fluid in muscles and joints, stiffening them the next day. Trainers now recommend a quick, cool shower rather than a luxurious hot tub.

Today, first aid for virtually any sports injury calls for cold, not heat. If professional treatment is not necessary, the home remedy is a combination of rest, ice, compression and elevation, often summarized by the mnemonic RICE.

Rest is the first, the most important—and the most often neglected—part of this therapy. Athletes who are injured should stop playing immediately. Those who pursue the mystique of "playing with pain" or "walking off" an injury almost always incur further harm; even if the pain does not immediately get worse, an injured muscle, tendon or ligament will suffer progressive damage from continued activity. Aggravating an injury in this way prolongs the healing process, and can lead to the formation of scar tissue that causes permanent weakness or disability.

Chilling is universally accepted as the essential second step. It numbs the pain and constricts blood and lymph ves-

sels to minimize swelling and inflammation. Immediately after the injury—on the field if possible—an injured limb should be soaked in 40° F. ice water for five to six minutes, massaged with ice molded inside a paper cup, or wrapped with a towel or a plastic bag full of crushed ice. The ice is left in place for about 30 minutes at a time, with at least 15 minutes between applications to allow the injured part to warm up; treatment is continued at least twice a day until swelling and tenderness disappear, usually three or four days after the injury. Applications of ice should be discontinued if they become painful.

Compression, with an elastic stocking or elastic bandage of the type that is available at drug stores, reduces swelling and usually is applied until the swelling goes down. The injured part is wrapped snugly, but not so tightly that blood circulation is cut off; if the compression causes pain, numbness or muscle cramps, it is too tight. Elevating the injured part—with a footstool, for example—helps drain fluid from the swollen area. Aspirin also helps to reduce both pain and inflammation.

Most injuries require no treatment other than the RICE program. But if the injured part swells alarmingly or if a visible bruise forms immediately, a doctor should be consulted within a few hours; a longer wait often allows valuable diagnostic signs to disappear and may delay recovery. Overuse injuries, which ordinarily are painful but produce no visible symptoms, require a physician's attention if pain persists for more than three to four days.

As injuries have grown more common, treatment has become much more sophisticated, and a number of physicians now specialize in sports medicine. When surgery is required, ingenious procedures devised to help professional athletes now improve the prognosis considerably (and have proved a boon to people hurt in household accidents as well). A few years ago, surgery routinely ended an athlete's career and might cripple him for life. Today, surgeons can mend injuries so well that the athletes return to the line-up later the same season. In one ingenious operation, carbon filaments are threaded in place of a ruptured ligament, providing a scaffolding for the regeneration of the injured cord; in an-

Watching on a screen (center background), a surgeon employs television as he mends a runner's knee without cutting the joint open. The assistant at right holds an arthroscope, a miniature TV-camera lens inserted into the knee through a tiny tube, while the surgeon removes damaged cartilage from the kneecap with a motorized shaver (inset), similarly inserted.

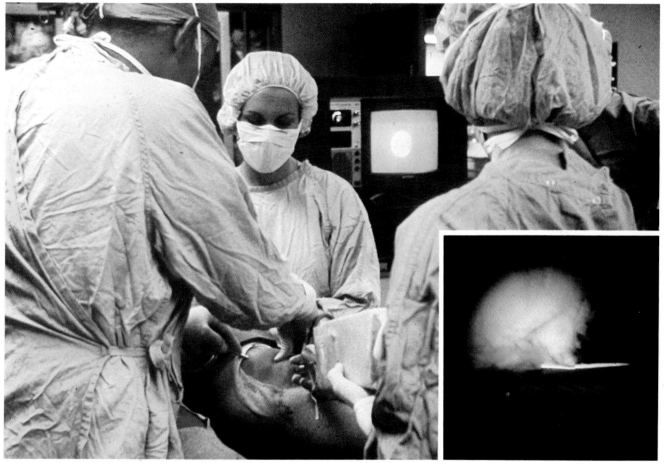

other, a transplanted tendon can replace a mangled ligament.

Rehabilitation after an injury begins as soon as the athlete leaves the operating room or the doctor's office. At first, most physicians prescribe a graduated course of stretching exercises, isometric exercises and "range-of-motion" exercises, in which the athlete moves the injured part through the air in each direction as far as he can without pain. After anywhere from two days to two weeks, the range-of-motion exercises are moved to a tub of water, which provides slight resistance. Later calisthenics and weight-training exercises are added, to strengthen the muscles and ligaments even as they knit together. And finally, when an athlete goes back

onto the field, compression bandages are used to provide extra support for the injured part and to prevent it from exceeding its natural range of motion—the reason that professional athletes are swaddled in tape for months after they return from an injury.

But of course prevention is better than any cure. In the sports that attract most amateurs, understanding and making use of the exercises that improve performance—the routines that train specific muscles for the strength, speed and flexibility that are needed for the unique actions of a sport—go a long way toward forestalling injury and making games the pleasure they are supposed to be. ❅

CHAPTER 5

The power that makes a muscle move

Fast twitches and slow twitches
The muscle engine
The ATP refinery
Long-term energy—the aerobic method

A hiker strides along a forest path. Scores of muscles in his arms, legs and trunk smoothly, rhythmically contract and relax. The muscle contractions supply the action that moves his body. The energy to contract the muscles comes indirectly from the food the hiker has eaten. Through a series of complex chemical reactions, his body has converted food into a special chemical, the only fuel that can directly power muscles, and another series of reactions has made the fuel give up the energy that produces motion.

How effectively this biochemical energy conversion—metabolism—is accomplished depends in part on the hiker's physical condition. If he is fit, not only does he have a stronger body and greater endurance than an unfit individual, but he also has a capacity for metabolism that can produce more energy for bodily functions. In fact, the overt signs of fitness—greater strength and endurance, for example—are outer manifestations of that more effective metabolism. Exercising to improve fitness accomplishes its goals mainly by increasing metabolic capacity. That is why efforts to promote fitness can be aided by an understanding of metabolism and of the principal site where it improves with training: the muscle.

Muscles, which are involved in all bodily functions that require movement—such as walking, running, breathing, talking, controlling blood flow and forcing food through the digestive system—exist in three basic types. The muscles used for body movement are generally under voluntary, conscious control. These are the skeletal muscles. The heart, automatically operated by the nervous system and ordinarily not under conscious control, is composed of another kind of tissue called cardiac muscle. A third type of tissue, called smooth muscle and also automatic, serves internal systems, propelling food through the stomach and the intestines and constricting blood vessels to adjust blood flow. For the most part, only the voluntary skeletal muscles benefit directly from exercise. Heart muscle is strengthened by endurance exercises, but this effect is secondary, the indirect result of increased demand on the circulatory system by the skeletal muscles. Skeletal muscles thus are the key to fitness.

Many of the more than 400 skeletal muscles can be seen outlined under the skin of lean people, but far more are hidden inside the body. They range in size from the large gluteus maximus of the buttocks to the small muscles that control such delicate functions as moving the eyelids.

Most skeletal muscles are attached to bones, thus the name. The attachment is indirect, through bands or cables called tendons; the ends of the muscles taper into the tendons, which connect to the bones. When the muscles act, they use the bones as levers to produce movement. Most are paired, one set in opposition to the other on opposite sides of a bone. For example, the biceps muscle, which lies on the front of the upper arm, flexes the elbow; the triceps muscle, lying along the rear of the same bone, straightens the arm out.

Muscles perform such motions by contracting, thus pulling on bones (or in some cases, tissues) to cause movement. The muscles always pull, regardless of the direction of the movement that results; when the arms or legs push against

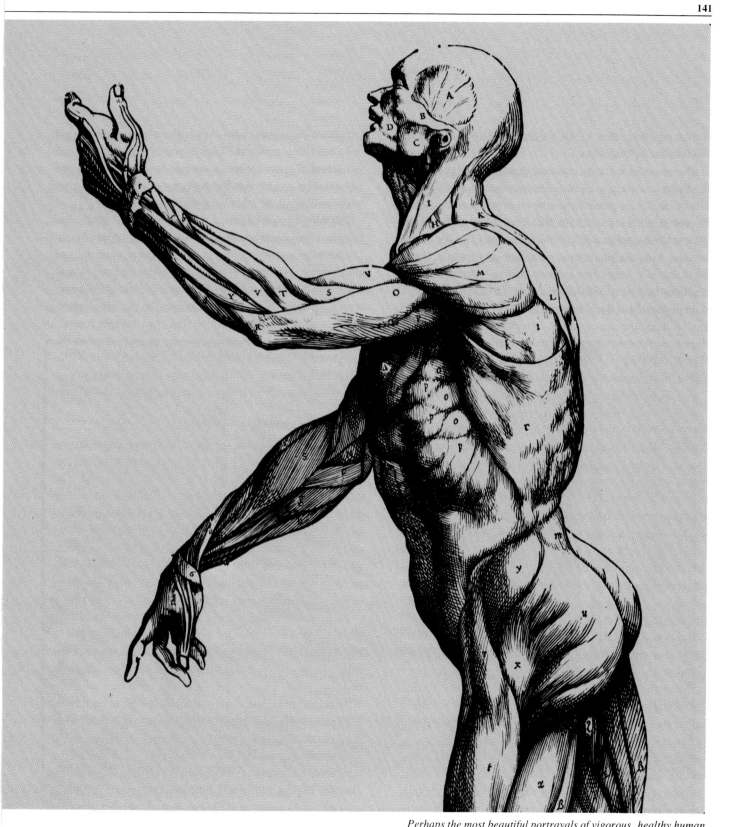

Perhaps the most beautiful portrayals of vigorous, healthy human muscles were also the earliest to depict them accurately. This example by an anonymous artist is one of the 277 illustrations for a revolutionary treatise on the structure of the body by the 16th Century Paduan physician Andreas Vesalius, who was the first to determine anatomy by the dissection of human cadavers.

ber of blood vessels around the fibers and causes connective tissue throughout the muscle to thicken, thus increasing muscle diameter.

The result of all these changes is muscles newly rich in myofilaments, with more cross bridges available to pull more actin filaments and produce more forceful contractions.

In addition to these structural improvements, changes in the muscles' control system can also be effected by exercise. One type of experiment, conducted with both human subjects and laboratory rats, has demonstrated that weight training of one arm or leg can produce strength gains not only in that limb but in the opposite one as well. This so-called cross transfer phenomenon apparently comes about because exercise forces the nervous system to ''turn on'' more fibers. When it learns to do so for muscle on one side of the body, it automatically does the same for the counterpart muscle on the other side. Support for this theory has come from other experiments comparing voluntary contractions with artificial, electrically induced contractions of muscle. The artificial contractions produce more force, suggesting that voluntary contractions leave some muscle fibers idle and that the nervous system can be made to turn on more of them.

The influence that the nervous system has on strength may explain why combat soldiers, weight lifters and martial arts competitors utter fierce screams and yells when maximum effort is necessary. The effect is more than psychological. Experiments at George Williams College in Chicago showed that a sudden loud noise such as a scream or a pistol shot produced momentary strength gains. Somehow the noise jolted the nervous system so that more muscle fibers were turned on than otherwise would have been.

These changes in nerve control and physical structure affect mainly the fast-twitch fibers, which are needed for anaerobic activities such as weight lifting and sprinting. The aerobic exercises that are so important to fitness depend on the slow-twitch fibers and also foster their development. The slow-twitch fibers, too, increase in size with exercise, partly because of the demand they place on the circulatory system. Calling for oxygen, they stimulate the growth inside the muscle of additional capillaries, the tiny blood vessels that deliver oxygen and nutrients directly to tissues.

One study found that there were, on the average, 1.5 capillaries per muscle fiber in trained muscle but only one per fiber in untrained muscle. As the muscles' work load increases, the capillaries apparently can no longer deliver as much blood as the muscles need. This brings about a localized shortage of oxygen and encourages new capillaries to grow into the oxygen-short areas.

The need for oxygen imposed by endurance exercise does more than stimulate the growth of additional blood vessels to increase the supply of blood. It also causes improvements in the chemical handling of the oxygen carried by the blood. The first clue to such exercise-related changes came from studies of hunting dogs. In 1926—long before muscle mechanisms were understood—Dr. George H. Whipple of the University of Rochester School of Medicine and Dentistry discovered that hard-working hunting dogs contained a higher concentration in their muscles of a substance called myoglobin than did dogs that were inactive pets. In 1934 grazing cattle were compared to penned-up cattle, with the same result. It is now known that myoglobin is the chemical that carries oxygen into the muscle cells. With more myoglobin, more oxygen becomes available and more aerobic work can be done—endurance increases.

The muscle engine

All the muscle changes that result from exercise—enlarged myofibrils, higher chemical concentrations, a more active nervous system—are interrelated. Each kind of improvement assists the others. Fundamentally all arise from alterations in the way the body generates the energy that makes the muscle mechanism operate. The muscle can be thought of as an engine. Like any other engine, it cannot work without fuel. An automobile engine converts the chemical energy in gasoline to mechanical energy. The muscle, with the help of the digestive, respiratory and circulatory systems, converts the chemical energy in food into mechanical motion.

But unlike an automobile engine, which uses fuel supplied to it directly, the muscle acquires usable energy by an indi-

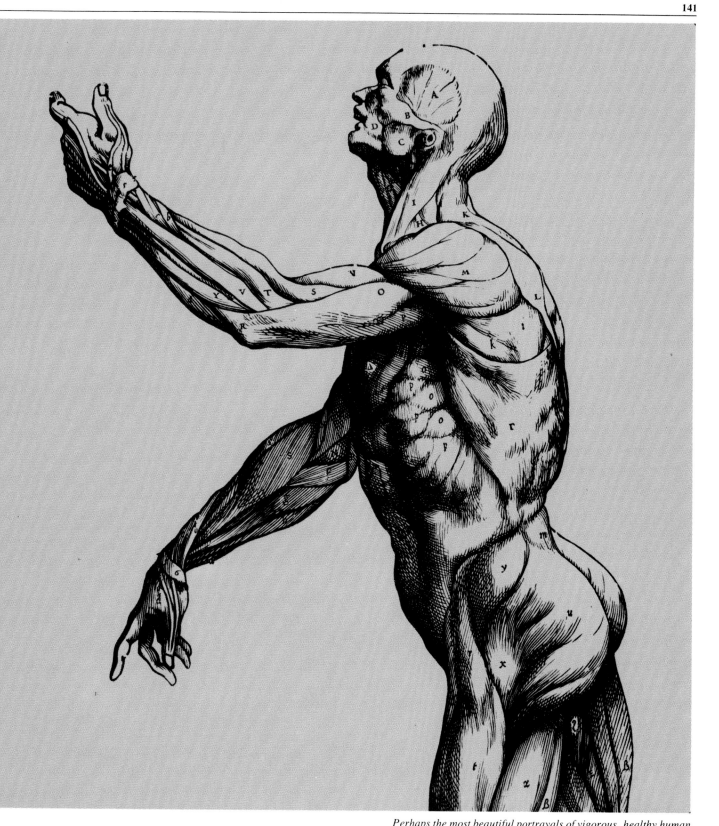

Perhaps the most beautiful portrayals of vigorous, healthy human muscles were also the earliest to depict them accurately. This example by an anonymous artist is one of the 277 illustrations for a revolutionary treatise on the structure of the body by the 16th Century Paduan physician Andreas Vesalius, who was the first to determine anatomy by the dissection of human cadavers.

something, their muscles are pulling on the bone levers to produce the pushing force.

That muscles work by contracting was first suggested in the Second Century A.D. by Galen, physician for the gladiators in ancient Pergamum and author of texts that dominated European medicine for more than a thousand years. Galen attributed the contraction to ''animal spirits'' flowing to the muscles from the brain through nerves—an idea that, if not taken literally, resembles modern theory—but later physicians outlined more outlandish notions. In the 17th Century, Alfonso Borelli of the University of Pisa thought that ''nerve gas'' inflated the muscles, then fermented to cause contraction. Borelli's contemporary, the English physician Francis Glisson, refused to accept the idea of nerve gas and maintained that the muscles responded only to irritation.

Not until 20th Century techniques of microscopy disclosed the composition of the muscles *(pages 158-165)* was it possible to arrive at a fairly complete description of the way they contract. The intimate views of skeletal muscle now available reveal that it is made somewhat like a child's Chinese boxes—a puzzle composed of successively smaller parts, one contained within another. In skeletal muscle, the parts are cylinders, each concealing inside it yet smaller cylinders.

The muscle is composed of cylindrical bundles and the bundles are made of cylindrical fibers—some as much as a foot long. Each fiber is a single cell enclosed in its own membrane, which acts as a gatekeeper, letting metabolic substances into and out of the cell. Each fiber is itself made up of hundreds of still-smaller cylinders called myofibrils.

Even the myofibrils are not the smallest part of the muscle. They also are divided—not longitudinally like the larger components, but crosswise—into minute cylindrical chambers known as sarcomeres. The sarcomeres, too, have parts. Extending inward from the ends of each sarcomere toward its center are slender threads called actin filaments. In the center of the sarcomere and extending outward toward each end, overlapping the actin filaments, are thicker threads called myosin filaments.

Although the mechanism that makes these parts contract has not been established with complete certainty, physiolo-gists have discovered what they believe to be the muscle's basic operating principle. They express it in what they call the sliding filament theory, according to which only the minuscule actin and myosin filaments in the sarcomeres do the work, pulling all the other components with them.

The thick myosin has many small projections, called cross bridges, extending outward like the bristles of a bottle brush. During muscle contraction, these projections reach out and attach themselves to the thinner strands of actin lying next to them, and then they pull. The two kinds of strands slide over each other in such a way as to shorten the muscle slightly. Next, in hand-over-hand fashion, the cross bridges release, grasp in a new position and pull once again to shorten the muscle more. During contraction, the actin and myosin filaments themselves do not shorten; they simply slide past one another so that they overlap more and more.

Fast twitches and slow twitches

This action can be made stronger, faster and longer-lasting by exercise, each type of exercise having an effect that depends principally on the kind of muscle fiber involved. The fibers in skeletal muscles come in two basic varieties; they differ in the rate at which they can convert fuel into mechanical energy. One kind is called fast-twitch, the other slow-twitch. As the name implies, the fast-twitch fiber contracts almost twice as fast as the slow-twitch. Fast-twitch fibers are the larger of the two and much paler, almost white, in color; slow-twitch ones are dark reddish-brown.

Each muscle contains a mix of the two. Understandably, most sprinters have muscles containing a greater number of fast-twitch fibers, while marathon runners have more of the slow-twitch variety. Such differences in numbers are probably inherited, and exercise does not seem to alter these differences as much as it does the effectiveness of each type.

Exercise generally increases the size of one type of fiber relative to the other; then the proportion of total muscle weight made up by one type may change, even though the number of each kind of fiber remains the same. In addition, exercise can alter chemical reactions and nerve impulses, again affecting one type of fiber more than the other. Jogging increases slow-twitch capacity, while sprinting or weight training increases fast-twitch capacity.

How these changes come about is now beginning to be understood. When a muscle is subjected to an exercise such as weight training, a probable outcome is an increase in size of the whole muscle. Such growth results, according to the most widely accepted theory, because the myofibrils making up the fast-twitch fibers increase in size and number. Training with weights, the theory suggests, requires such strenuous contractions that the covering around the myofibrils stretches, opening up pores to let in more nutrients—particu-

larly amino acids, the building blocks of the protein molecules that form all kinds of muscle tissue. The increased supply of amino acids can then be used to make protein for additional actin and myosin filaments inside the myofibrils, expanding the size of the myofibrils. Some myofibrils may grow so much that they divide, creating entirely new ones. The result is an increase in the bulk of myofibrils and thus of the size of the fibers that the myofibrils form—and finally of the muscles that the fibers form.

Scientists agree that muscle growth has more than one cause. They believe that weight training increases the num-

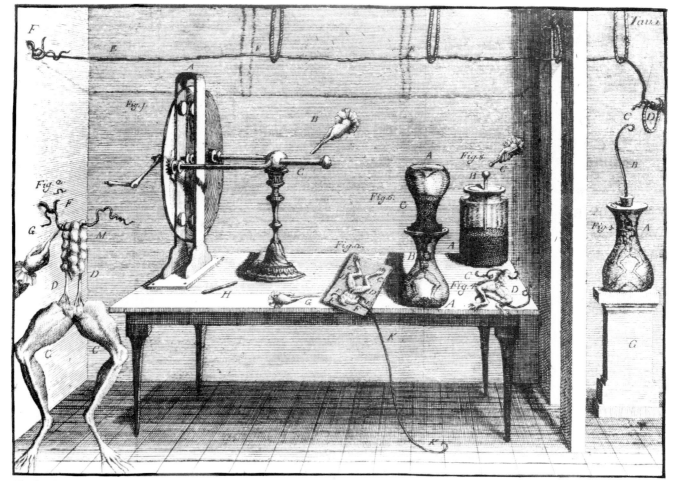

The hand-cranked static-electricity generator in this 18th Century engraving was used by Italian anatomist Luigi Galvani in the 1780s to prove that electrical nerve impulses stimulate muscle action. Applying voltages produced by the generator to freshly dissected frogs' legs (left), Galvani caused the legs to twitch.

ber of blood vessels around the fibers and causes connective tissue throughout the muscle to thicken, thus increasing muscle diameter.

The result of all these changes is muscles newly rich in myofilaments, with more cross bridges available to pull more actin filaments and produce more forceful contractions.

In addition to these structural improvements, changes in the muscles' control system can also be effected by exercise. One type of experiment, conducted with both human subjects and laboratory rats, has demonstrated that weight training of one arm or leg can produce strength gains not only in that limb but in the opposite one as well. This so-called cross transfer phenomenon apparently comes about because exercise forces the nervous system to "turn on" more fibers. When it learns to do so for muscle on one side of the body, it automatically does the same for the counterpart muscle on the other side. Support for this theory has come from other experiments comparing voluntary contractions with artificial, electrically induced contractions of muscle. The artificial contractions produce more force, suggesting that voluntary contractions leave some muscle fibers idle and that the nervous system can be made to turn on more of them.

The influence that the nervous system has on strength may explain why combat soldiers, weight lifters and martial arts competitors utter fierce screams and yells when maximum effort is necessary. The effect is more than psychological. Experiments at George Williams College in Chicago showed that a sudden loud noise such as a scream or a pistol shot produced momentary strength gains. Somehow the noise jolted the nervous system so that more muscle fibers were turned on than otherwise would have been.

These changes in nerve control and physical structure affect mainly the fast-twitch fibers, which are needed for anaerobic activities such as weight lifting and sprinting. The aerobic exercises that are so important to fitness depend on the slow-twitch fibers and also foster their development. The slow-twitch fibers, too, increase in size with exercise, partly because of the demand they place on the circulatory system. Calling for oxygen, they stimulate the growth inside the muscle of additional capillaries, the tiny blood vessels that deliver oxygen and nutrients directly to tissues.

One study found that there were, on the average, 1.5 capillaries per muscle fiber in trained muscle but only one per fiber in untrained muscle. As the muscles' work load increases, the capillaries apparently can no longer deliver as much blood as the muscles need. This brings about a localized shortage of oxygen and encourages new capillaries to grow into the oxygen-short areas.

The need for oxygen imposed by endurance exercise does more than stimulate the growth of additional blood vessels to increase the supply of blood. It also causes improvements in the chemical handling of the oxygen carried by the blood. The first clue to such exercise-related changes came from studies of hunting dogs. In 1926—long before muscle mechanisms were understood—Dr. George H. Whipple of the University of Rochester School of Medicine and Dentistry discovered that hard-working hunting dogs contained a higher concentration in their muscles of a substance called myoglobin than did dogs that were inactive pets. In 1934 grazing cattle were compared to penned-up cattle, with the same result. It is now known that myoglobin is the chemical that carries oxygen into the muscle cells. With more myoglobin, more oxygen becomes available and more aerobic work can be done—endurance increases.

The muscle engine

All the muscle changes that result from exercise—enlarged myofibrils, higher chemical concentrations, a more active nervous system—are interrelated. Each kind of improvement assists the others. Fundamentally all arise from alterations in the way the body generates the energy that makes the muscle mechanism operate. The muscle can be thought of as an engine. Like any other engine, it cannot work without fuel. An automobile engine converts the chemical energy in gasoline to mechanical energy. The muscle, with the help of the digestive, respiratory and circulatory systems, converts the chemical energy in food into mechanical motion.

But unlike an automobile engine, which uses fuel supplied to it directly, the muscle acquires usable energy by an indirect route. The muscle cannot use roast beef, mashed pota-toes and ice cream for fuel. Food must first be converted by the digestive system into simpler substances that can be used by the muscle engine. In the muscle the energy inherent in these simpler substances is extracted to build a chemical called adenosine triphosphate—ATP—which is the only fuel the muscle can use directly.

ATP is a rather complex assemblage of chemical groups. The central part of its molecule is adenosine—which itself is a combination of two substances, adenine and a form of sugar called ribose. Attached to the basic building block of adeno-sine are three phosphate groups, each composed of one atom of the element phosphorus and four atoms of oxygen.

That phosphate compounds have something to do with living energy was recognized in the early 1900s. But not until the 1940s was the mechanism fully explained, principally by two German-born refugees from the Nazis. ATP was estab-lished by Dr. Fritz Lipmann as the unique compound that supplies energy for all life—not just muscular action in hu-mans but also cell division, digestion, growth and all the

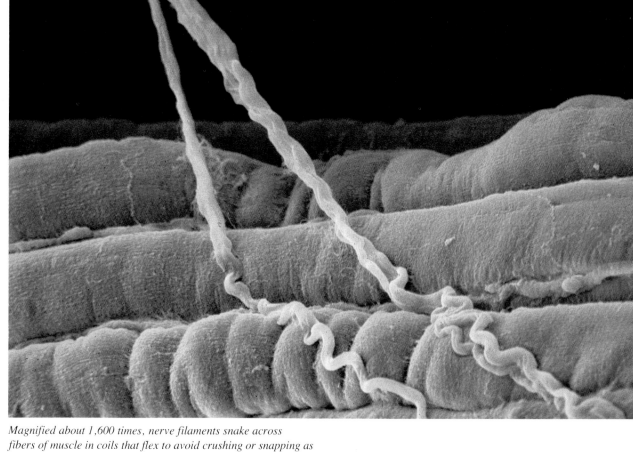

Magnified about 1,600 times, nerve filaments snake across fibers of muscle in coils that flex to avoid crushing or snapping as the fibers contract and relax. Each filament delivers its actuating signals to a terminal called a motor end plate (not shown), which is located on a single muscle cell.

processes of life in all plants and animals. Lipmann accomplished his work at one after another of the most famous research centers of Europe and America, including the Biological Institute of the Carlsberg Foundation in Copenhagen, the University of Heidelberg, Massachusetts General Hospital in Boston, Harvard Medical School, and Cornell University Medical College and The Rockefeller University in New York City.

How the body is kept supplied with ATP by a complex cycle of chemical reactions was discovered by Dr. Hans Krebs, who fled Germany for England and did most of his work at Oxford. He and Dr. Lipmann shared the Nobel Prize in Physiology and Medicine in 1953, and Dr. Krebs was knighted by Queen Elizabeth II in 1958.

The critical parts of the ATP molecule are the bonds holding the phosphate groups to the adenosine center. Energy is required to form such connections, and that energy is released when the bonds are broken. The phosphate groups are attached in the ATP molecule by bonds that contain exceptionally large amounts of energy; when one such bond is broken, much of this energy is released and becomes available to make sarcomere filaments pull on each other and contract muscles.

The intricate process that enables ATP to power movement begins in the brain. When it orders a muscle to move, a nerve impulse travels down through the spinal cord and through a nerve to the muscle that the brain has selected. When this signal, a ripple of electrical and chemical activity, reaches the muscle fiber, it triggers a chain of reactions. The first reaction changes the permeability of the membrane surrounding each fiber. This allows atoms bearing a positive electrical charge—positive ions—to flow through the membrane from the surrounding fluid.

This incursion of positive ions alters the delicate chemical and electrical balance of the muscle cell, setting off another wave of reactions that ultimately changes the shape of protein molecules bound to actin. It uncovers receptor sites into which the myosin molecules can fit exactly, like pieces of a jigsaw puzzle fitting into each other. Electrical attraction between the two brings them together, and when myosin fits

into its matching site in the actin, the myosin snaps like a released spring, changing its shape. That snap of the myosin pulls the actin filament with it, shortening the sarcomere and contracting the muscle. A crucial step in this sequence is the snap releasing the "spring" of the myosin molecule—a spring originally set by ATP.

After the cross bridge has been moved by the snap of the myosin spring, an ATP molecule attaches itself to the myosin and breaks the linkage between myosin and actin. Now a stimulating chemical at one end of the myosin molecule, an enzyme called ATPase, can begin working. The enzyme breaks the connection of one of ATP's powerful phosphate groups. That sets the spring. When the myosin fits into an actin site, the spring snaps and energy is released to move the cross bridges. The remains of the ATP molecule—a phosphate group and a molecule of adenosine diphosphate (ADP)—come free.

This process continues so long as the nerve signal continues and ATP is supplied. Actin's receptor sites are uncovered, myosin fits in, the myosin spring snaps to release energy and contract the muscle, the debris is dropped, and then a fresh ATP molecule is picked up by the myosin to set the spring once again. This action, in which the sarcomere becomes shortened as the actin and myosin filaments pull on each other in a hand-over-hand motion, can be repeated hundreds of times in the course of a one-second contraction.

Eventually, the brain stops giving the signal for the contraction. At that point, the chain of reactions is interrupted, the breakdown of ATP halts and no more energy is released. The myosin cross bridges let go of the actin filments, and the sarcomeres lengthen to their original relaxed positions.

The complex action of the muscle contraction is an all-or-none process. A stimulated muscle fiber contracts either fully or not at all. It cannot produce graded amounts of force. Of course the whole muscle can produce anything from a gentle caress to a jaw-cracking uppercut. The differences in force arise from the differing numbers of fibers that are activated, not from the extent to which each one is activated.

And yet, despite the all-or-none action of muscle fibers, the system acts with astonishing precision. Even the simple

Charting the hot spots of a hard-working body

At the Laboratory for Aerobiology in Harrow, England, scientists used an electronic device known as a thermographic camera to gauge variations in skin temperature of runners before and during exercise.

The eerie pictures *(right)* confirmed what physiologists had already discovered with more primitive techniques: Skin temperature, on the average, is lower during exercise than at rest—sweating makes the skin pass heat more quickly to the surrounding air than it does ordinarily. But the pictures also revealed something new. Skin that covered muscles used for running was warmer than skin elsewhere on the body, suggesting that heat is passed directly from the working muscles through the skin to the air.

Furthermore, this effect was most pronounced in runners with little or no fat between muscle and skin to impede the transfer of heat. The researchers concluded that fatter runners rely more on blood flow to carry heat from the muscles and distribute it over a wider area of skin. This effect can deprive muscles of blood during exercise and may limit the runner's speed and endurance.

Skin Temperature (Fahrenheit)

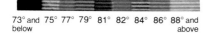

73° and 75° 77° 79° 81° 82° 84° 86° 88° and
below   above

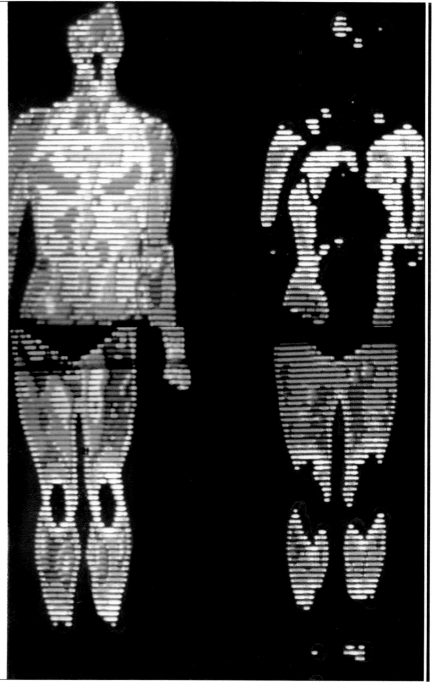

Heat pictures of a long-distance racer before a run (right) and just after (far right) show changes in skin temperature, as indicated by the color code above. Before running he is warmer than after—sweat has cooled the torso from blue and yellow to black. But the thighs and shins, where heat from hard-working muscles has radiated through the skin, have turned blue-green— the warmest temperature on the scale.

matter of standing upright requires the delicate interplay of huge numbers of fibers. Groups in the large muscles of the trunk aided by scores of muscles in the feet and legs maintain posture as they repeatedly contract and relax to maintain just the proper tension to resist gravity.

In some cases, the skeletal muscles perform feats of balancing without conscious commands from the brain. Consider, for example, someone standing on the deck of a rolling boat. As the angle of the deck changes, the pattern of nerve impulses going to thousands of motor units is constantly adjusted. A continuously changing pattern of muscle forces is generated in various groups of muscles to precisely counterbalance the force of gravity in a changing situation.

Think also of the exquisite patterns of neural and muscular activity going on as a virtuoso violinist plays a dazzling passage, or as a tennis player leaps into the air, simultaneously twisting his body, looking over his shoulder, and reaching upward and outward to hit a ball traveling at high speed in a direction different from his own. Neither the violinist nor the tennis player gives any thought to the orchestrated symphony of actions and reactions going on within his body. Each simply wills his body to perform certain motions, and the body handles the details.

The ATP refinery

To power these intricately coordinated actions of nerves, chemicals and tissues, the body must have ATP, the only fuel muscles can use. Yet the amount of ATP in the body is very small. Instead of being held in reserve, ATP is largely manufactured as needed. In this way the body is analogous to the diesel locomotive. This type of locomotive is made to move not by energy generated by the diesel engine itself. Rather, the engine turns an electrical generator. The generator produces electricity, which then powers electric motors that drive the wheels. Thus the fuel that turns the wheels—electricity—is not kept available in storage for use, but is made as needed from another kind of fuel that can be stored. The body does much the same thing with ATP, but in a more complicated way.

When ATP releases energy, it does so by letting go of one

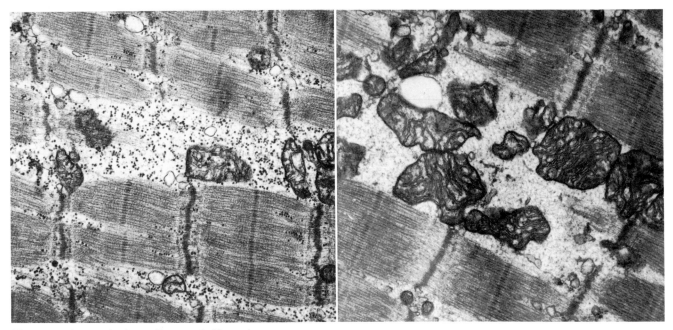

These two microscopic views of leg muscle fiber, taken from the same man before exercise and after, show how activity uses glycogen, the sugar substance that supplies energy to the body. Before working to pedal a bicycle, the muscle is stocked with black specks of glycogen (left); after exercising for 100 minutes, the exhausted muscle contains almost no glycogen.

of its three phosphate groups. When that happens, ATP becomes ADP, adenosine diphosphate, a molecule with two rather than three phosphate groups. ADP is made back into ATP by energy harvested from food. This energy reattaches the phosphate group that had been split off, regenerating ATP so that the cycle of ATP to ADP to ATP can continue and the power latent in food can be transferred and realized in muscular action.

The diesel locomotive has only one way of making the electricity it needs. The body, by contrast, has numerous methods of making ATP for the muscles. Each method involves a different series of chemical reactions, but there are only two fundamentally different kinds. One kind is aerobic, requiring oxygen to proceed; and the other is anaerobic, operating without oxygen. Differences in processes make some methods better suited than others for particular purposes.

Just as exercises can be selected to develop specific muscles for specific activities, so can muscles be trained to produce energy more effectively by specific methods for specific purposes. Football players generate their energy largely by one method, distance runners by another. To improve, each must train the method that will be involved. Thus an understanding of the methods for energy transfer in the body is helpful in planning an exercise program.

The anaerobic methods can operate for only a relatively short time—they are used principally in the fast-twitch muscle fibers—but some work longer than others. The fastest and most quickly exhausted of these processes for regenerating ATP, called the speed system, makes use of the energy in a phosphate compound that already exists within the muscle: creatine phosphate. The bond holding the phosphate group to the creatine is split by an enzyme, releasing energy. That energy is then used to reattach the freed phosphate onto ADP, turning it into ATP.

The muscle contains a relatively small amount of creatine phosphate, which must be produced in the fibers when they are at rest. There is perhaps enough for six to eight seconds of all-out exertion, and it cannot be replenished until the exertion halts for about a minute. Yet this small supply is enough for sprinting a few yards for a bus or dashing up a flight of stairs. The short bursts of activity powered primarily from the creatine phosphate reservoir are also critically important in certain sports. Football and many track-and-field events depend on this mechanism. Its effect on the 100-yard dash, for example, is apparent during the last few seconds of such a race. By then the reservoir of creatine phosphate is depleted and the runners begin to slow down. The winner is usually the one who slows down the least.

Because the creatine phosphate supply is so limited, vigorous activities that must go on for longer than a few seconds need ATP produced from a more plentiful raw material. In the main anaerobic method, the intermediate system, which can produce fresh ATP for two or three minutes, the raw material is glucose, often called blood sugar. Glucose is made by the body from the carbohydrate foods, such as bread, pasta and beans. Most glucose is then converted into a kind of starch called glycogen, which can be stored and converted back to glucose as needed. Some glycogen is kept in the muscles, and some is held in reserve in the liver.

When vigorous exercise begins and the muscles use up their immediately available stores of creatine phosphate, they begin breaking down their stored glycogen. Meanwhile the liver also begins converting its glycogen to glucose, which is transported to the muscles by the blood. In the muscles both glucose and glycogen are acted on by several enzymes in an extremely elaborate series of chemical reactions that finally yield, as one of their products, the ATP needed to fuel muscular contraction. This anaerobic process proceeds very rapidly and is important in such sports as sprinting and sprint swimming.

Although the anaerobic production of ATP with the glucose and glycogen reactions is useful because it can generate quick energy, it cannot continue for very long because of the by-products that come out of the processes along with ATP. The most important are hydrogen and a substance called pyruvic acid. As excess hydrogen atoms build up they combine with pyruvic acid to form lactic acid, the acid in milk. The lactic acid is carried rapidly away from the muscle by the bloodstream. But if the strenuous activity continues, the blood cannot remove lactic acid rapidly enough and its concentration in the muscle will rise. According to one theory, the increasing acidity slows ATP production by inhibiting the chemical reactions that extract energy from glucose. The result is a progressively more severe feeling of fatigue, and eventually exercise must stop.

Long-term energy—the aerobic method

Although the metabolic methods that operate without oxygen are important, they are severely limited both in the amount of energy they can extract from the available materials and in the length of time they can generate energy. The aerobic method, on the other hand, cannot produce energy at as fast a rate as the anaerobic processes, but it can continue for extended periods of time, and it can extract a very large part of the energy contained in raw materials that are stored by the body in plentiful supply.

The aerobic process, like the important anaerobic one, can work with glucose, and the early stages of the process are identical. Glucose is broken down to pyruvic acid, releasing energy to make ATP. Then comes a major difference. Because oxygen is available, pyruvic acid does not combine with hydrogen to form lactic acid. Rather, the oxygen enables special enzymes to convert pyruvic acid into a crucial intermediary called acetyl-CoA, which will then produce still more ATP by a process that also yields hydrogen atoms and carbon dioxide gas. The carbon dioxide is carried away by the blood as waste. The hydrogen combines with oxygen, producing water for the blood to dispose of and eventually releasing large amounts of energy to synthesize ATP.

The waste products of this aerobic process—water and carbon dioxide—are one of its advantages. They are easily excreted by the body and do not build up in the muscle fibers to cause fatigue, as does the lactic acid generated anaerobically. But the great value of an aerobic method is the cycle of reactions—called the Krebs cycle after its discoverer, the Oxford biochemist Dr. Hans Krebs—that follows the initial breakdown of glucose and the conversion of pyruvic acid into acetyl-CoA.

The Krebs cycle takes place deep within the muscle cell, inside sausage-shaped compartments, called mitochondria, around the myofibrils making up each fiber. It is a very efficient mechanism because it is a cycle—a lengthy sequence of reactions that ends up by re-creating the same substance needed to start it. This substance is yet another of the many acids involved in metabolism, one named oxaloacetic acid. It reacts with acetyl-CoA, producing other substances that react with one another, to produce still others and so on and on. The final step reconstitutes oxaloacetic acid, which can start the cycle over again by going to work on a fresh molecule of acetyl-CoA. Along the way from oxaloacetic acid back to oxaloacetic acid, the cycle spills out the crucial by-products: some ATP and a lot of hydrogen atoms.

This freeing of hydrogen is particularly important. The hydrogen eventually combines with oxygen from the blood to make water, by a long, complicated process. At several stages of this process, it releases the large amounts of energy needed to make more ATP. The result is very efficient production of ATP. The raw materials and their by-products are repeatedly worked over within the muscle until all the chemical energy contained in them has been extracted and employed to rebuild ATP molecules or turned into heat. Because of this efficiency, the aerobic process makes available almost 200 times as much muscle energy as anaerobic ones.

The efficiency of the chemical reactions in aerobic metabolism is only one reason why this process can produce so much energy. Equally important is its ability to draw upon a number of different raw materials. Unlike the principal method of anaerobic metabolism, which can take energy only from the glucose made from carbohydrate foods, the aerobic system can use fats and proteins as well. It converts the molecules that are linked together in protein—amino acids—and fats into the acetyl-CoA needed to keep the Krebs cycle going.

Thus the muscular engine is less like a diesel locomotive, which must have diesel oil to run, than it is like a utility steam boiler that can burn either coal, oil, gas or processed garbage. The muscles can even use several raw materials simultaneously, adjusting the mix as the intensity and duration of the exertion demand more or less energy.

For any activity—even getting up out of a chair—the

The powerhouse inside a muscle

When a tennis player returns a serve, or a bean shoot breaks through the soil, or a firefly lights up, or a student works out a math problem, each is doing biological work. To do it, they use the only chemical that directly supplies biological energy — adenosine triphosphate, or ATP. This life-sustaining substance consists of a backbone of atoms in a structure called adenosine, to which are attached three groups of phosphate, each containing the element phosphorus linked to oxygen atoms and to the other groups by high-energy bonds. Only about three ounces of ATP exist in the human body at any one time, but it is continuously created, consumed and re-created. The ATP a student uses for an hour of homework is minute; it could be replaced with the energy derived from a few peanuts. If the student spends an hour playing tennis, he might use as much as 10 pounds of ATP — in tiny bits,

made, unmade and remade in his muscles throughout the hour.

The methods by which the muscles make ATP, diagramed in the following pages, depend on the demands that must be met. Taken together, these methods somewhat resemble the conduct of a war. First the store of ATP already available, like a forward outpost, is engaged and almost immediately lost. The muscles call for support, synthesizing ATP from a small supply of a substance called creatine phosphate, which can briefly meet the challenge until more energy can be brought to bear. These front-line energy sources give the body time to summon reserves by a process that produces ATP rapidly but inefficiently *(page 154).*

If the demand continues, mobilization of all the body's resources provides steady, moderate and enduring energy by the process called aerobic metabolism *(overleaf).*

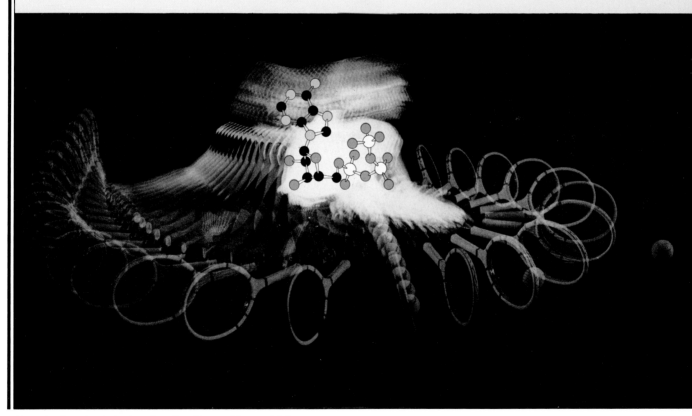

A tennis champion's forehand stroke, dissected in a multiple-exposure photograph by Harold E. Edgerton, is powered by adenosine triphosphate, whose molecule is superimposed in the model at center. Three phosphate groups project to the right from the adenosine backbone: The yellow balls are phosphorus atoms; the red, oxygen; the blue and black, nitrogen and carbon.

For the long haul, aerobic metabolism

To keep a jogger running for miles or a swimmer going for many laps, the muscles consume so much ATP that this compound must be continuously replaced through an efficient and enduring process: aerobic metabolism. This process produces the energy to reconstitute ATP by using oxygen, supplied by the lungs and carried in the blood, and a variety of raw materials derived from food. It can extract most of the energy available in food, and it does so without leaving behind any toxic by-products.

The aerobic method of restoring ATP molecules draws mainly on the food energy in carbohydrates and fats, but it can also make some use of proteins. These food materials, broken into simpler compounds in the digestive system and further refined in the liver and other organs, enter into a long sequence of reactions inside the cells of the muscle tissue. Along the way, some energy is released to rebuild ATP, but most of the energy is produced by a complicated cycle of many reactions (*following pages*).

The process presents an apparent paradox. Though it is named after oxygen, it makes no direct use of the element until the last of its many reactions, when oxygen combines with hydrogen to form water, one of two ultimate waste products; the other is carbon dioxide. But the paradox is not real. Oxygen's role is not simply that of sanitation. As it picks up hydrogen refuse, the oxygen completes a chain of chemical transformations that releases a final jolt of energy for ATP synthesis.

GETTING ENERGY OUT OF ATP
The source of all living energy, ATP (right, top), links adenosine and three phosphate groups (P) by electrochemical bonds. When a muscle needs energy, the outermost bond (red zigzag line) is snapped off (center) by a chemical activator, or enzyme, releasing the power of the broken bond for use by the muscle. For such continued exertion as running—first analyzed photographically (below) by Eadweard Muybridge—ATP molecules broken up this way are reconstituted by aerobic metabolism.

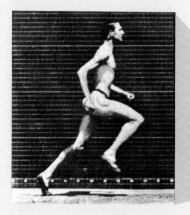

PUTTING ENERGY BACK INTO ATP
To keep the muscles working, the bond that broke to release energy must be restored and the phosphate group that was snapped off must be put back, reconstituting the ATP molecule (near right). When the energy to perform this rebuilding is supplied by the aerobic method, it is extracted step by step from nutrients in food, as outlined in the block diagram opposite.

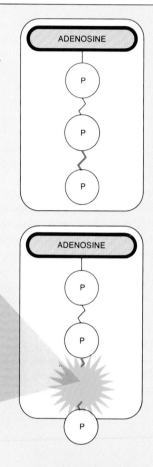
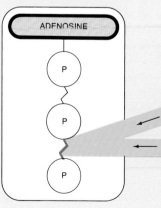

PYRUVIC ACID

Aerobic metabolism starts with a breakdown of carbohydrates that yields some energy for ATP along with pyruvic acid. This first reaction does not require oxygen.

ACETYL-CoA

Pyruvic acid, fats and proteins are changed into a substance called acetyl-CoA, which is essential to the next stage of aerobic metabolism.

THE KREBS CYCLE

Acetyl-CoA and substances derived from protein pass through a sequence of reactions named the Krebs cycle after its discoverer, biochemist Sir Hans Krebs. The cycle produces some energy for making ATP, gives off carbon dioxide as a waste product and pulls hydrogen atoms out of a changing chemical mix.

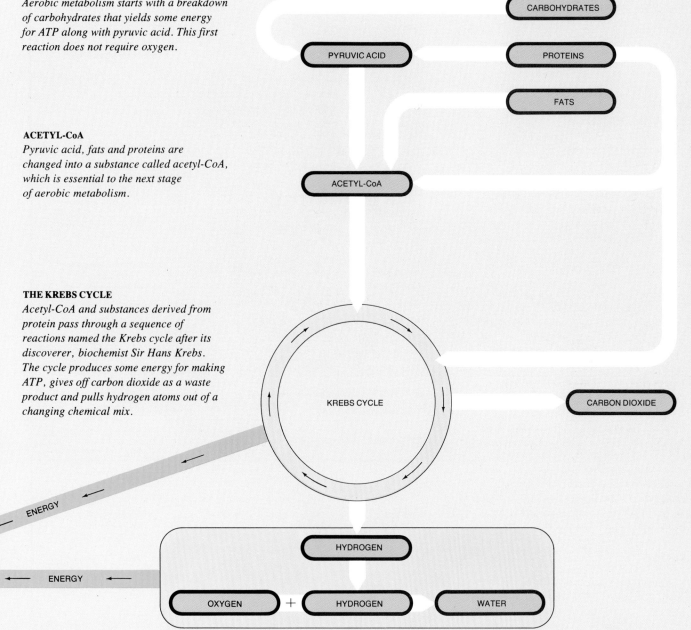

OXYGEN AND HYDROGEN

In the final phase of aerobic metabolism (yellow rectangle, bottom), the hydrogen from the Krebs cycle enters into chemical reactions that release great amounts of energy for the resynthesis of spent ATP. Eventually, oxygen combines with the hydrogen, yielding water as a final waste product.

For spurts of energy, anaerobic metabolism

Quick, vigorous effort—even the simple task of getting up out of a chair—uses energy faster than the aerobic process can provide it. The diagrams on this page show other ways of reconstituting ATP—anaerobically (without oxygen). These processes are more responsive, though less efficient.

CREATINE PHOSPHATE
For instant energy, the muscles draw on a small supply of a compound called creatine phosphate. Split by an enzyme when the body makes a sudden effort, it releases the power of its own phosphate bond to re-create ATP—but in less than 10 seconds the supply is gone.

CARBOHYDRATES
If the demand continues, anaerobic energy production gets under way, using carbohydrates to generate ATP. But this is a profligate process: It consumes carbohydrates at a tremendous rate and extracts less than 6 per cent of their energy.

PYRUVIC ACID
The end product of the breakdown of carbohydrates is pyruvic acid. This stage of the anaerobic process also releases hydrogen, which combines with the pyruvic acid in the muscles to form lactic acid.

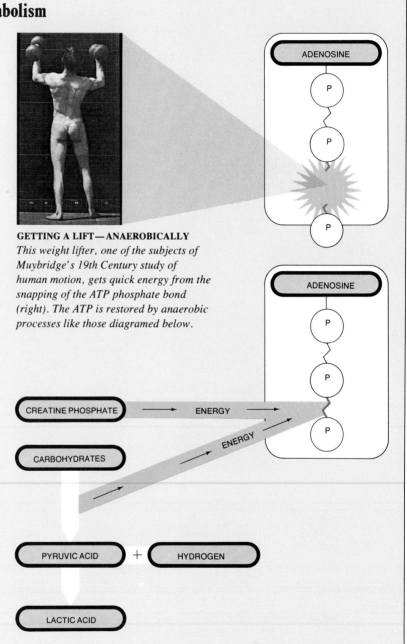

GETTING A LIFT—ANAEROBICALLY
This weight lifter, one of the subjects of Muybridge's 19th Century study of human motion, gets quick energy from the snapping of the ATP phosphate bond (right). The ATP is restored by anaerobic processes like those diagramed below.

LACTIC ACID
The lactic acid builds up in the muscle despite the best efforts of the blood to remove it. Lactic acid produces a feeling of fatigue; eventually, according to one widely accepted theory, it interferes with the muscle's ability to keep making ATP.

muscles first generate energy from the tiny store of ATP already on hand. That lasts no more than a few seconds. For the next few seconds, the raw material is creatine phosphate. Before it, too, is gone, conversion of the muscles' own supply of glycogen has begun to provide energy. All of these processes are anaerobic and depend only on materials previously stored in the muscles. Still, they can power the muscles for a minute or two—enough for an 800-meter race or a 200-meter swim.

Meanwhile, some aerobic metabolism has been supplying energy for the heart, lungs and other organs. If exertion is continued for more than a few minutes, aerobic metabolism is called upon to support it as well, using glycogen mainly from the slow-twitch fibers and glucose from the bloodstream. Extended activity is supported by a gradually increasing consumption of fats. After a half hour of jogging or swimming, fats contribute roughly half of the energy, but over an hour or two they can supply up to 80 per cent. It is easy to see why prolonged exercise is so effective in getting rid of body fat. The supply of fat in a well-fed person is almost impossible to use up, however; in a man of average size who is not overweight there is enough fat to supply the energy for running 600 miles.

Although carbohydrates and fats supply most of the raw materials for aerobic metabolism, proteins are also used, but only in very small amounts—unless an individual is starving or exercises strenuously for several hours, as in running a marathon. Then he must consume some of the protein making up his own muscle tissue in order to keep going.

The anaerobic threshold

In the body's automatic adjustment of the mix of raw materials being used to produce energy, the changeover between aerobic metabolism and anaerobic metabolism is the key to endurance. When there is no effort at all—as when someone is sitting quietly in a chair—the body must of course operate aerobically to keep its essential organs working. Almost any additional effort, however, starts up the fast anaerobic processes. The body will switch back to long-lasting aerobic metabolism if the effort required can be sustained by that process. Almost anyone can maintain a slow walk aerobically for a long time but he may not be able to keep up a faster pace that way; then the body turns toward anaerobic metabolism and fatigue quickly increases. The higher the level of work that can be sustained before this threshold is reached, the greater the endurance, for with a high threshold, strenuous exertion does not require inefficient anaerobic metabolism.

The threshold depends on the body's maximum ability to make use of oxygen—VO_2max. For most people, the anaerobic threshold comes at about 60 per cent of VO_2max. At that point the demand for oxygen exceeds the body's ability to supply it. That is why a high VO_2max increases endurance—it raises the anaerobic threshold.

Still, someone whose VO_2max is only moderate can perform feats of endurance provided he restricts the level of exertion, always keeping his energy expenditure below the limit set by his modest anaerobic threshold.

A 32-year-old woman applied for entry into the New York Marathon several years ago, thinking that in the five months before the race date she would have plenty of time to transform herself from a casual jogger into a long-distance runner. But as the months passed, distractions kept her from training regularly. One week she got in perhaps six miles of running, the next week 15, and once in a while, 20. Some weeks she did not run at all.

Two days before the marathon, she had the traditional pre-race spaghetti dinner with a group of friends who were entered in the race—but then she decided that she herself would not run. On race day, when she went to see her friends start the marathon, she changed her mind; she began the race to see how far she could get before having to give up and take a bus to the finish to meet her friends.

Five hours 25 minutes later, she crossed the finish line, tired but not exhausted. She had kept her pace well below her anaerobic threshold. And while sporadic training had left her with a low VO_2max and low anaerobic threshold, she ran slowly enough to avoid the anaerobic metabolism that would have generated fatigue-causing lactic acid, and thus she was able to keep going for the full 26 miles 385 yards.

Of course most marathon runners—even those with high VO₂max and high anaerobic thresholds—finish as tired and winded as anyone else who exerts himself nearly to capacity. Explanations for these aftereffects are beginning to come out of the research laboratories.

The reason for extreme muscle fatigue among those who exercise aerobically was a mystery, because aerobic metabolism does not generate the lactic acid that may cause exhaustion in anaerobic activity. One solution to the mystery was proposed by David Costill, Director of the Human Performance Laboratory at Ball State University.

In 1972, using studies done earlier in Sweden, Costill and his colleagues examined runners in a 30-kilometer race.

They took samples of muscle tissue from their subjects at the end of the race. The slow-twitch and fast-twitch muscle fibers were examined under a microscope and then each type of fiber was analyzed for its content of glycogen. The muscles' glycogen, derived from carbohydrate foods, is one of the sources of energy that regenerates ATP by both aerobic and anaerobic metabolism. The researchers found that although the fast-twitch fibers from their runner subjects still held ample glycogen reserves, the glycogen in the slow-twitch fibers was essentially depleted. They concluded that when the slow-twitch fibers have used up their stores of glycogen, the fast-twitch fibers are unable to carry the load for long. Distance runners thus feel fatigued when their slow-

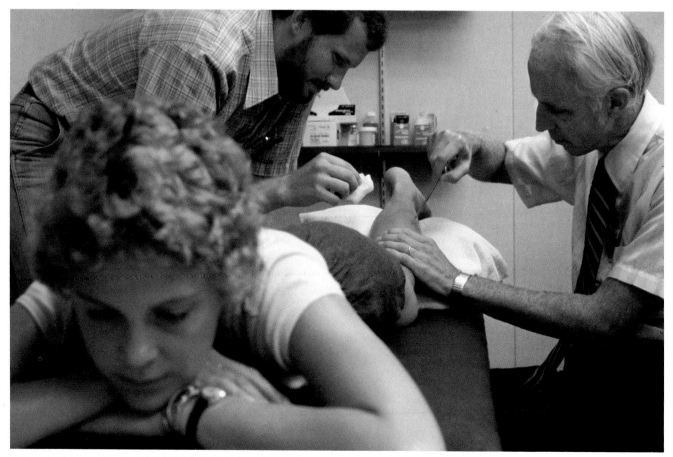

Using a hollow needle, David Costill of the Ball State University Human Performance Laboratory samples muscle tissue from an athlete's anesthetized calf. Analysis of such specimens—about the size of a grain of rice—reveals the ratio of two types of muscle fibers that act at different speeds (opposite) and allows Costill to guide athletes toward sports suited to one type or the other.

twitch fibers no longer have a supply of glycogen, even though other parts of their muscles may still hold a considerable amount of glycogen.

Even if exercise is not carried to exhaustion, however, it takes a toll on the body. The most familiar symptom is the one that is graphically described as "being out of breath." The body is indeed low on oxygen, and the supply is not readily replenished. When the exercise stops, breathing does not return to the normal rate immediately. If the exercise was not strenuous, the recovery period is short. But if the exerciser was working very hard—running all out for several blocks, for instance—he might gasp and breathe heavily for a prolonged period before his breathing returns to normal. This happens because the metabolic methods involved in generating energy create what is known as an oxygen debt, and the kind and extent of the debt depend on the methods that were used.

A person exercising at a moderate rate—say, walking briskly—incurs a modest oxygen debt. In the early stages of the exercise, his oxygen consumption and breathing rate rise fairly rapidly until he is providing enough oxygen to support the aerobic reactions going on in the muscles. His body is then meeting its energy needs by the aerobic method. So long as he maintains aerobic metabolism, he does not run up a large oxygen debt. But during the brief period when his breathing rate was still rising, he did. Aerobic metabolism

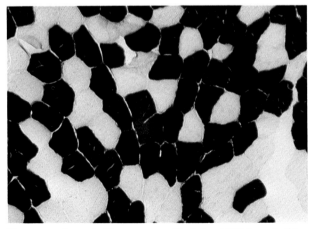

Two types of muscle fiber are magnified about 100 times in this cross section of tissue from a human thigh. The stained segments are fast-twitch fibers, which give short bursts of energy and are usually larger than the light-colored slow-twitch fibers. However, in this muscle, strenuous bicycle exercise has enlarged the slow-twitch fibers to about the same size as the others.

lagged slightly behind the energy demand, so some of the energy he needed was produced anaerobically. His creatine phosphate stores were drawn down a bit, and a small amount of lactic acid accumulated.

When the walk ends, his breathing and heart rates remain somewhat elevated for a short period; they must, so that the body can continue producing energy at slightly above a resting rate to recharge the ATP and creatine phosphate supply, and get rid of the small amount of lactic acid. Because the contribution from the anaerobic sources was small, his recovery is rapid. Half of the total oxygen debt is repaid within 25 to 30 seconds, and his breathing returns to normal in one or two minutes.

The oxygen debt is much greater and takes longer to repay if the exercise is more strenuous. If a person is walking up a long, steep hill, aerobic metabolism cannot supply enough energy, and anaerobic sources are called on to turn out energy at a high rate. Lactic acid is produced rapidly and accumulates in the muscles and blood. Now, not only does his ATP and creatine phosphate supply have to be recharged, but some of the lactic acid generated during this intense work will have to be converted back into glucose in the liver, a process that requires oxygen.

These functions take substantially longer than does the recovery from light exercise, for a number of reasons not directly connected to the exercise itself. The respiratory muscles involved in heavy breathing must themselves work hard and thus use a lot of oxygen. The heart muscle must work hard, too, and because a great deal of heat is generated by muscles in converting the chemical energy of food into mechanical work, body temperature increases. Higher temperature speeds all of the body's metabolic processes. And the faster metabolism calls upon the respiratory system for still more oxygen.

Repaying the oxygen debt is the body's means of returning to a healthy equilibrium. Every time an individual incurs and repays an oxygen debt through exercise, he resets that equilibrium to a higher level—a reminder that he is paying off another obligation as well, his obligation to himself to keep fit. ❋

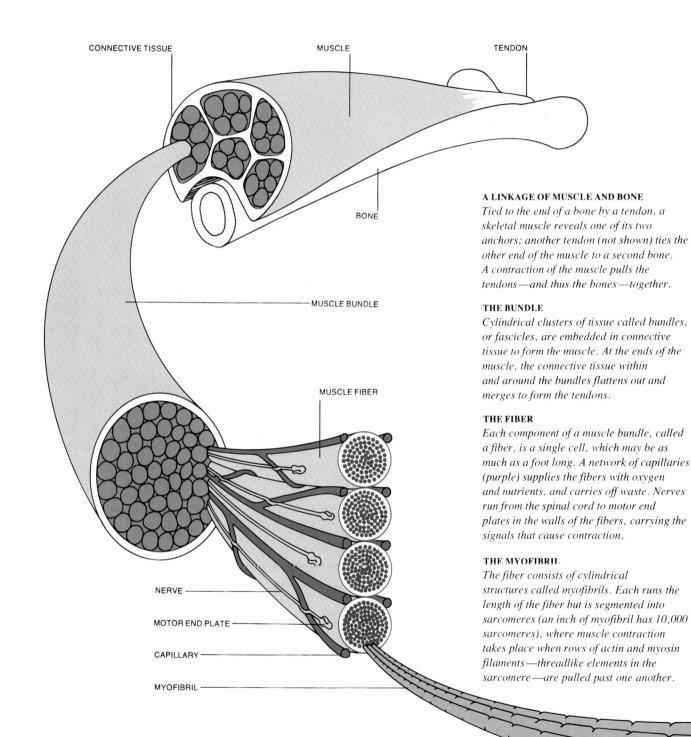

CONNECTIVE TISSUE

MUSCLE

TENDON

BONE

MUSCLE BUNDLE

MUSCLE FIBER

NERVE

MOTOR END PLATE

CAPILLARY

MYOFIBRIL

A LINKAGE OF MUSCLE AND BONE
Tied to the end of a bone by a tendon, a skeletal muscle reveals one of its two anchors; another tendon (not shown) ties the other end of the muscle to a second bone. A contraction of the muscle pulls the tendons—and thus the bones—together.

THE BUNDLE
Cylindrical clusters of tissue called bundles, or fascicles, are embedded in connective tissue to form the muscle. At the ends of the muscle, the connective tissue within and around the bundles flattens out and merges to form the tendons.

THE FIBER
Each component of a muscle bundle, called a fiber, is a single cell, which may be as much as a foot long. A network of capillaries (purple) supplies the fibers with oxygen and nutrients, and carries off waste. Nerves run from the spinal cord to motor end plates in the walls of the fibers, carrying the signals that cause contraction.

THE MYOFIBRIL
The fiber consists of cylindrical structures called myofibrils. Each runs the length of the fiber but is segmented into sarcomeres (an inch of myofibril has 10,000 sarcomeres), where muscle contraction takes place when rows of actin and myosin filaments—threadlike elements in the sarcomere—are pulled past one another.

Taking a muscle apart

A flexed muscle such as the magnificent specimen at right looks like a single homogeneous unit. It is nothing of the kind. Under the skin lies an almost unreckonably complex assemblage of parts, each part itself an assemblage of smaller and still smaller parts.

Identifying these parts has represented a triumph of modern science comparable to the geographical discoveries of the great Age of Exploration. The tool of discovery has been the microscope. The extraordinary photographs on the following pages show the components of a muscle with a depth and clarity attainable only with the most powerful version of the tool, the scanning electron microscope. (The tissues are from laboratory rats, but human muscle is almost identical.)

How the components fit together is depicted in the drawing at left, designed as a guide to the photographs. It represents the parts of a typical skeletal muscle—the kind that is attached to bones and powers the movements of exercise and sport. Some parts belong to the circulatory and nervous systems: capillaries that deliver fuel and remove waste, nerves that transmit messages from the brain. Others are unique to muscle and make it a complete power plant whose intricate machinery converts raw fuels into mechanical energy.

The sequence of this dissection of a muscle's parts begins with the component called a bundle, big enough to be seen by the naked eye; the photographs then take up the story. Ending the sequence is the infinitesimal unit called the sarcomere *(pages 164-165)*. The sarcomere does all the work. It has one function, and one only: to contract from an elongated, resting state to a shortened, stressed state. In millions of these minuscule contractions lies the true source of a muscle's power.

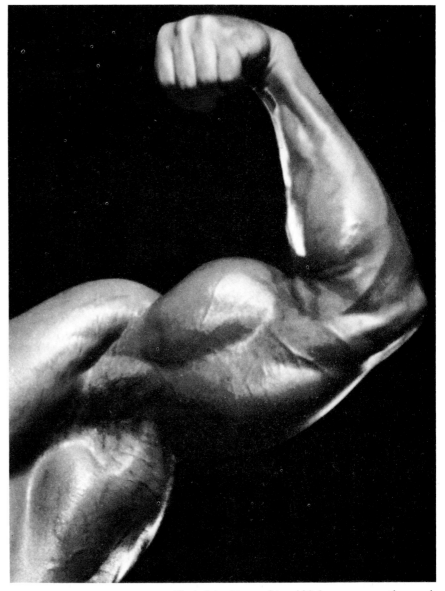

The bulging biceps of Arnold Schwarzenegger, the muscle builder who won the Mr. Universe title five times, represents an epitome of male muscle. Large muscles and great strength generally go together in men, although not necessarily in women.

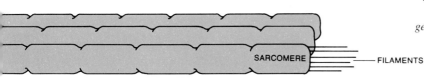

SARCOMERE — FILAMENTS

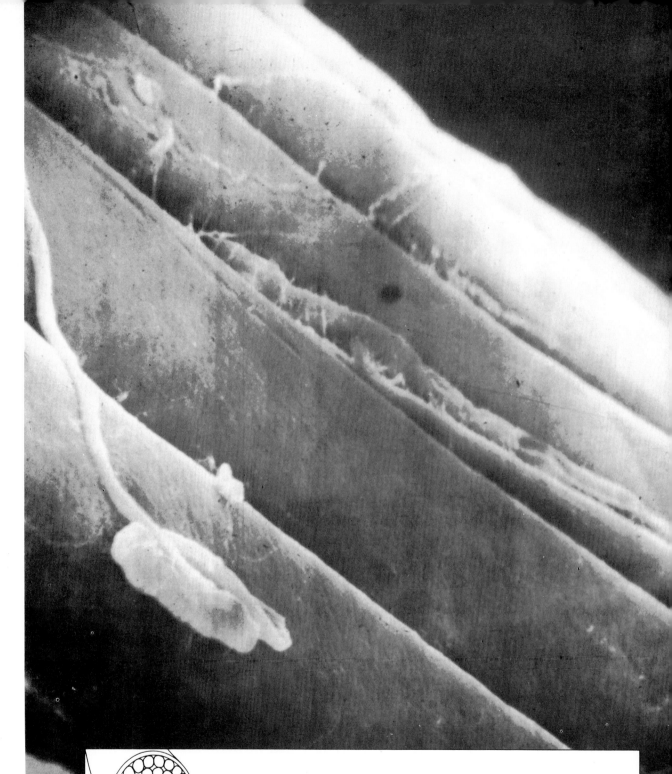

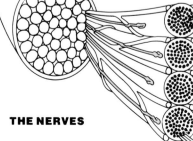

THE NERVES

The view above of part of a muscle—four fibers are visible —shows a tendril of nerve called an axon, making contact with a fiber at a motor end plate (foreground). The electrical signals that travel from the brain to the end plate through the nerves (green in the drawing at left) produce an action potential in the fiber—a change in electrical charge that triggers chemical reactions, ending in the release of energy. As few as 10 or as many as several thousand muscle fibers may be linked to one nerve cell to form a motor unit, where all fibers are activated at once.

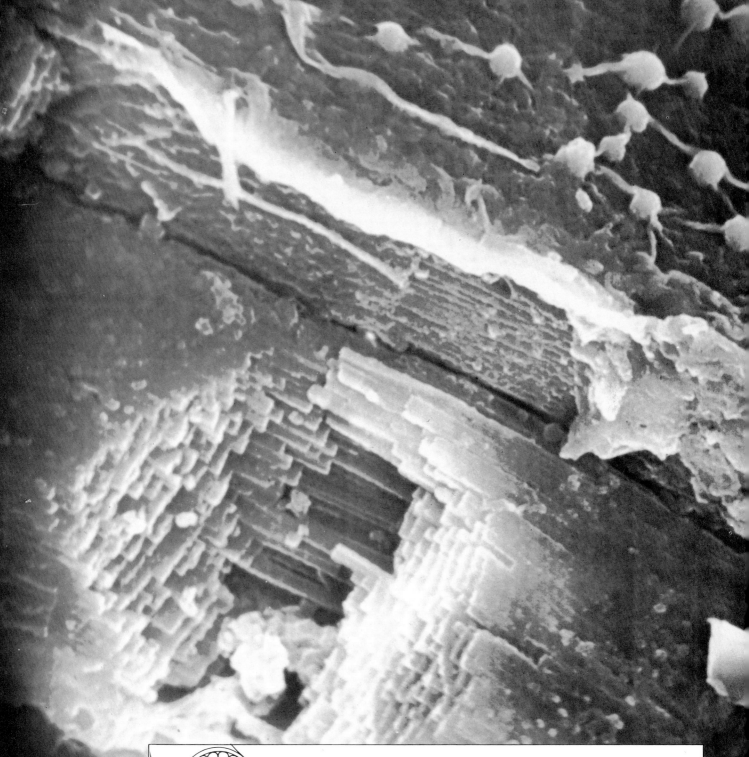

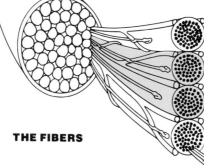

THE FIBERS

In this photomicrograph of two muscle fibers (shown in pink in the diagram at left), the fiber at bottom has been scooped out to reveal the long, thin myofibrils that make up the fiber; the fiber at top, coated with a network of remnants from the membrane that surrounded it, is intact. Fibers may be arranged either diagonally or parallel to the length of the muscle. Muscles with diagonal fibers contract more powerfully than those with parallel fibers, but over a shorter distance. About three fourths of the body's skeletal muscles are the diagonal-fiber type.

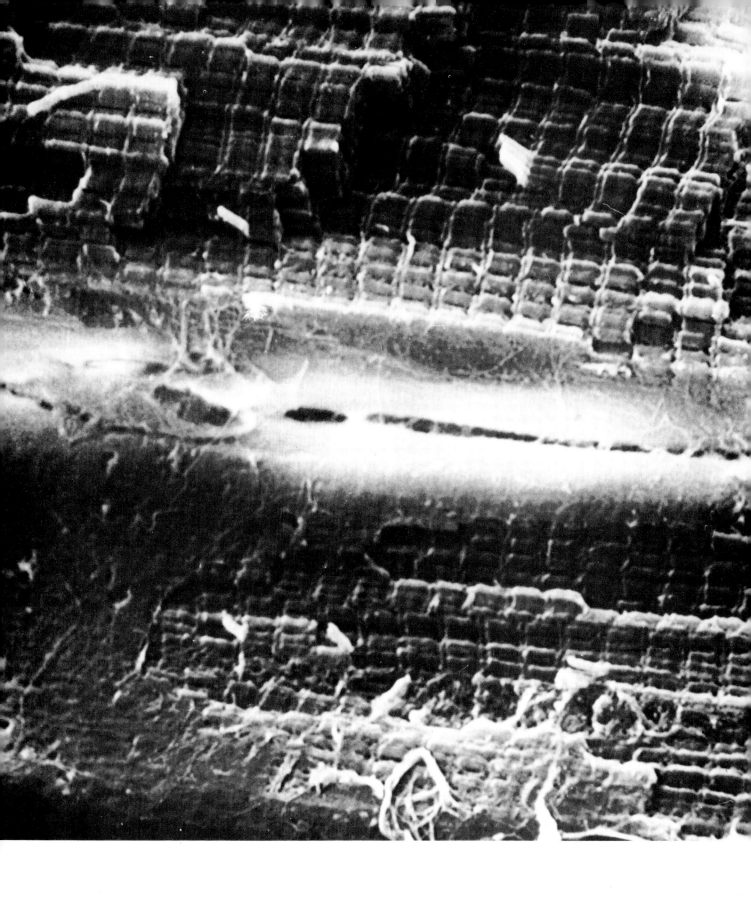

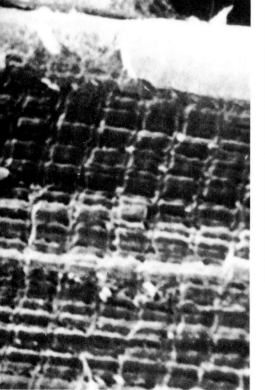

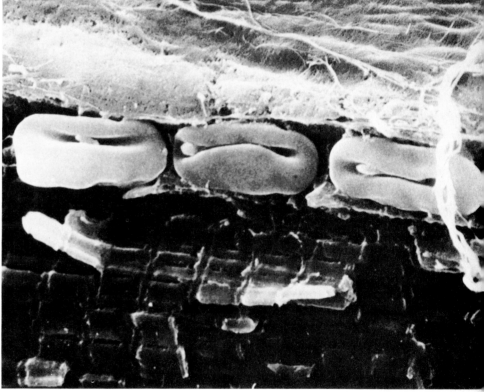

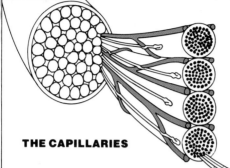

THE CAPILLARIES

Photomicrographs of pairs of fibers show capillaries (purple in drawing at left), which supply chemicals for the muscle's reactions and take away the wastes from those reactions. In one view (far left) a capillary has been cut on a slant to show its lumen, or bore. In the view below, three red blood cells squeeze through a capillary between two fibers. Their flat shape offers the greatest possible contact with the wall of the capillary, permitting efficient transfer of nutrients and wastes between fiber and blood.

164

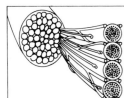

THE SARCOMERES

The photomicrograph below reveals the parts of muscle that do the work. The vertical lines, called Z bands, divide the myofibril into sarcomeres; the horizontal lines in the sarcomeres are the filaments that pull on one another (bottom). In the cross section at right, enlarged still more, the gridlike patches are Z bands, and the tiny dots filaments. The large dots are glycogen, a nutrient; the sausage-shaped bodies—mitochondria—process nutrients.

HOW A SARCOMERE CONTRACTS

In a relaxed state, a sarcomere and its filaments are extended; the thick myosin filaments in the center slightly overlap the thin actin filaments extending from the ends.

Myosin

Actin

RELAXED SARCOMERE

Using fuel from the mitochondria, tiny projections of the myosin — cross bridges — grab the actin filaments, pull, then let go. The filaments slide over one another.

Cross bridge

PARTIALLY CONTRACTED

Each cross bridge repeatedly engages an actin filament, swings, detaches and returns until the actin and myosin filaments almost completely overlap one another and the sarcomere is fully contracted.

CONTRACTED

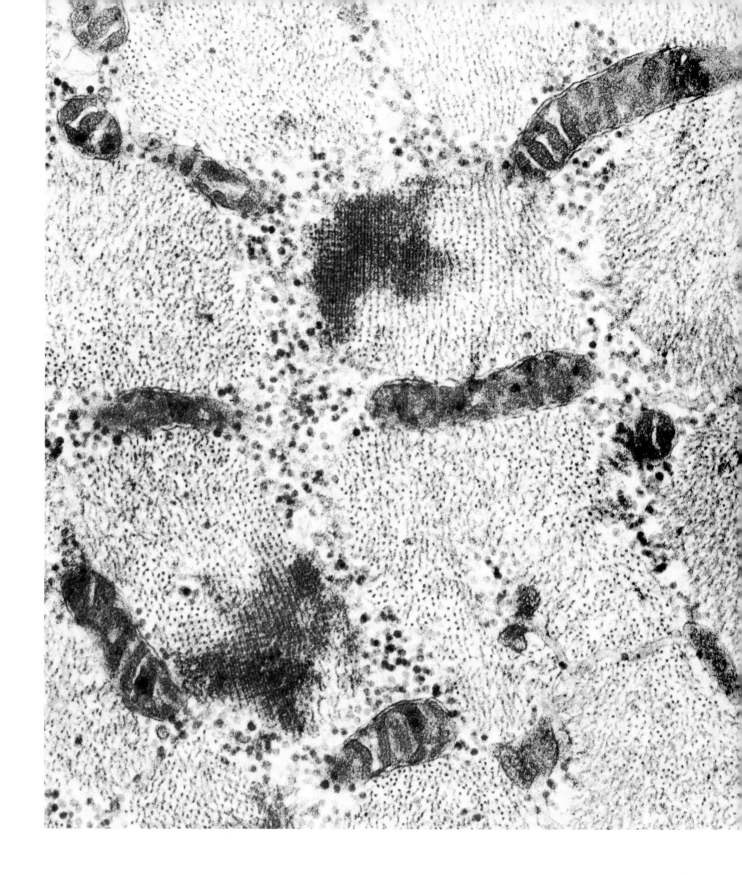

people beginning to exercise strenuously. The heart rate slows and the beat steadies when you end the exercise session, and the fluttering disappears entirely as fitness improves.

● **An uncomfortably rapid and wildly fluctuating heartbeat** that comes on in a sudden rush during exercise and subsides only after considerable rest may be a sign of ARRHYTHMIA. It may be harmless but it may also indicate heart trouble; if you experience arrhythmia even after reaching a high level of fitness, consult a physician.

● **A slower-than-normal resting pulse rate** is common among those in especially good physical condition. In such people, a heart rate below 60 beats per minute at rest is a good sign and no cause for alarm; it indicates a heart muscle with plenty of reserve strength.

HEART TROUBLE: *See CHEST PAIN*
HEAT EXHAUSTION: *See SKIN CHILLED AND DAMP*
HEAT PROSTRATION: *See SKIN CHILLED AND DAMP*
HEATSTROKE: *See SKIN DRY AND HOT*

HEEL PAIN. Pain under the heel bone may be due to a simple bruise caused by exercising in thin-soled shoes on hard surfaces or on surfaces containing sharp rocks and pebbles. A bruise should need only several days of rest to heal.

If pain under the heel spreads along the bottom of the foot or is accompanied by a bump either on the bottom of the heel or at the point where the heel meets the Achilles tendon, you may have PLANTAR FASCIITIS, a tear and inflammation of the tissues called fasciae, which protect nerves and muscles. Rest, soaking in warm water and massage are the best treatments; if the pain persists, consult a foot doctor. This ailment is caused by pressure, pounding or a sudden unexpected turn, and it can generally be prevented by well-cushioned and flexible shoes *(pages 76-77)*.

HEEL SPUR OR BUMP: *See HEEL PAIN*
HEEL TENDON PAIN: *See ACHILLES TENDON PAIN*

HIP PAIN. Few types of pain are as varied in degree or origin as those of the hip. Pain can be localized or can radiate from either or both of the hips into the lower back or down the leg, and it may originate from problems located outside the hip — in the lower back or in the knee, leg or foot.

● **Hip pain that radiates from the hip** to the back of the thigh and leg, often called SCIATICA, may be due to an unstable lower spine or to a ruptured spinal disc. Pain from these causes may be relieved by rest; if it persists, consult a physician.

● **Hip pain that is felt upon any motion,** usually with tenderness over part of the hip, is generally caused by inflammation. Apply an ice pack to the hip at least twice a day for 30-minute periods,

allowing 15-minute intervals between applications. You may apply the ice pack as often as you wish. If pain and swelling persist after one or two days of treatment, consult a physician.

● **Hip pain that is felt only when the hip is bearing weight,** especially in running, is generally caused by a STRESS FRACTURE. Do not run until pain in the foot and hip is relieved. If pain is still severe after a week, consult a physician.

● **Hip pain in the hip opposite to the one bearing weight** may result from a minor difference in the lengths of the legs, or it may be caused by a knee injury.

If you have hurt your knee and pain and swelling have not gone down after several hours, consult a physician. The hip pain can be relieved only by correcting the knee problem.

If you have not hurt your knee, compare leg lengths by standing erect in your bare feet while someone places his hands, palms down, around the crests of your pelvic bone; the hand on the shorter side will be seen to be lower. If you see such a difference, consult a physician for an accurate measurement and, if necessary, a prescription for a shoe heel lift to compensate.

● **Hip pain that is present only during exercise** is generally caused by FLAT or OVERPRONATED FEET *(page 137),* which roll the ankle inward. Shoes with arch supports may relieve the pain; if they do not, consult a foot doctor, who can prescribe a removable shoe support called an orthotic to correct the balance of your feet.

HYPOTHERMIA: *See SPEECH SLURRING*

INDIGESTION: *See STITCH IN THE SIDE*
INFECTION: *See SKIN IRRITATION and SKIN SCRAPES*

ITCHING FEET. Itchiness, scaling and dryness, usually beginning in the spaces between the third and fourth toes and sometimes spreading to the soles, signal athlete's foot, an infection by a fungus called ringworm. In hot weather the ailment may flare up into red, cracking, painful sores; infected toenails may become thickened and distorted in shape. Apply fungicide containing micronazole nitrate or undecylenic acid, available at drugstores. If you are susceptible to this fungal infection, take steps to keep it from attacking you in the first place. Do not walk barefoot in a swimming-pool area or locker room, where the disease is easily transmitted. Keep your feet as dry as possible by exposing them to air and by powdering them regularly with talcum powder. Always dry your feet thoroughly after bathing, and change socks frequently.

If athlete's foot resists home treatment, consult a physician. The fungus infection sometimes proves difficult to eradicate, and it may be complicated by bacterial infection.

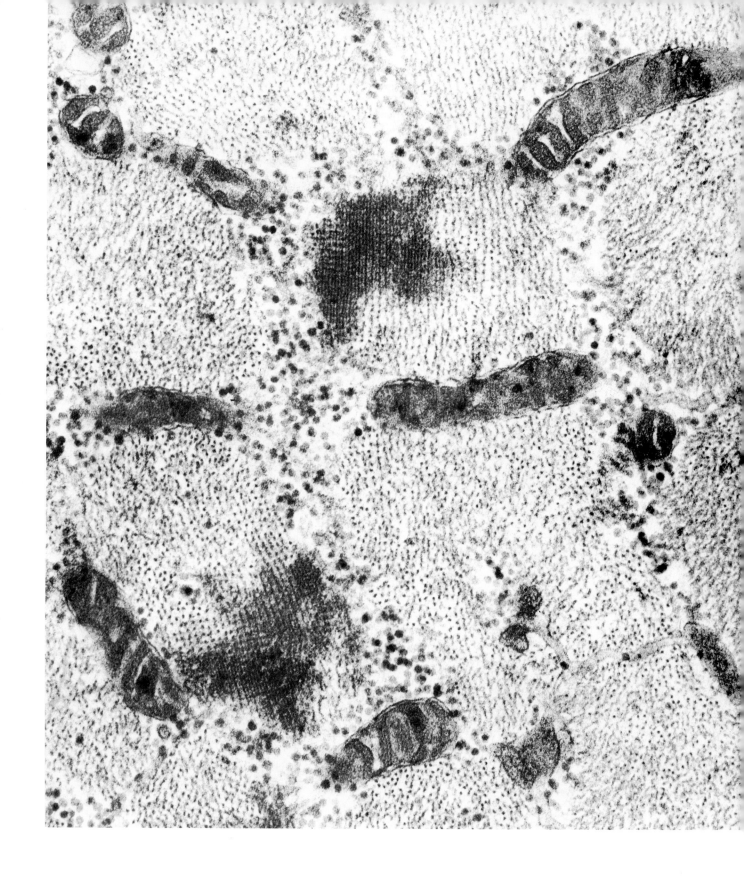

An encyclopedia of symptoms

Exercise is supposed to benefit health, not harm it, but it inevitably brings the risk of injury. Most injuries that do occur are minor and can be treated at home, but some are life-threatening emergencies that demand immediate medical care. When trouble strikes, it is vital to know when to rush to the hospital, when to wait to visit a doctor the next day, and when to treat the condition yourself. The most common indications of injury or disorder are described below, listed alphabetically by symptoms that can be felt or seen. The disease or injury that causes each symptom or group of symptoms is named in small capital letters.

ABRASION: *See SKIN SCRAPES*

ACHILLES TENDON PAIN. Pain and swelling at the back of the ankle, arising either during or after exercise, is generally due to inflammation of the tendon there; this condition is called ACHILLES TENDINITIS. Stop exercising and rest your leg until the pain and swelling begin to disappear. Aspirin relieves the pain, as do the shoe inserts called heel lifts: Do not walk barefoot or in flat-soled shoes or sandals. When pain and any swelling have been substantially reduced, start exercising regularly each day, increasing intensity and duration gradually. A lack of arch support can aggravate or even bring on tendinitis, and extra supporting inserts in your shoes may prevent a recurrence.

If home treatment does not relieve Achilles tendinitis, consult a physician at your convenience.

If pain is extremely severe and the leg is completely immobilized, you may be suffering from a RUPTURED TENDON. Consult a physician immediately.

ALLERGY: *See SKIN IRRITATION*

ANKLE PAIN. If ankle pain is sharp at first but later becomes dull, and if the ankle swells, then shrinks, you probably have a SPRAIN, caused by the tearing of the ligaments in the joint. Immediately apply four first-aid treatments, sometimes summarized as RICE: rest, ice, compression and elevation. Wrap a towel around your injured ankle and prop it up. Then apply a bag filled with ice cubes to the ankle. Caution: Do not place ice directly against the skin; it can cause pain. Now bind the ice pack and ankle together with an elastic bandage, available at drugstores, taking care not to wind the bandage so tight that you shut off the blood supply; the joint will become numb if you do so. When the bandage and ice pack have been in place for 30 minutes, unwrap the area and leave the skin exposed for 15 minutes to warm it. Then apply the ice pack again

and rewrap. Continue to use the sequence of bandage, ice pack and elevation at least twice a day for three to four days or until the swelling goes down; you may repeat the sequence as often as you wish. If the pain and swelling are not greatly reduced by that time, consult a physician.

If ankle pain steadily worsens and the swelling does not go down after several hours, you may have an ankle FRACTURE. Consult a physician immediately.

ARRHYTHMIA: *See HEART IRREGULARITY*
ATHLETE'S FOOT: *See ITCHING FEET*

BACK PAIN. Chronic low back pain, one of the most long-lasting and painful exercise problems, has a variety of causes, ranging in severity from a muscle strain or ligament sprain through differences in leg length *(see HIP PAIN),* to a ruptured spinal disc.
● **Relatively mild back pain that responds to rest and gentle massage** is probably muscle strain or ligament sprain. Either can usually be treated in the same way. Do not exercise until the pain disappears completely — generally a week or two — and when you start again, ease into your exercise routine gradually. Both conditions can be prevented by thorough warm-ups and by preseason exercises designed to condition the body. Sleeping with a bed board between the mattress and the box spring also helps prevent back pain. Do not sleep on your stomach; this position can cause a sway-back posture, which contributes to back pain.
● **Severe pain that radiates down one or both legs** may indicate that a RUPTURED SPINAL DISC is pressing on the sciatic nerve, which extends from the base of the spine down the thigh. Consult a physician immediately.

BLISTER. When repeated rubbing of the skin damages underlying tissues, body fluids accumulate to repair them, creating the sensitive, liquid-filled swelling of a blister. Blisters are an almost inevitable consequence of activity, until the skin toughens, and they cause serious harm if they become infected.
● **A small, uninfected blister** does not require treatment so much as protection against further irritation. Cover it with an adhesive bandage. The swelling should subside in two to three days.
● **A very puffy blister** will heal faster if you puncture it to let the fluid escape. Wash your hands thoroughly, and swab the blister and surrounding area with rubbing alcohol, which serves as an antiseptic. Sterilize a needle by holding it in a match flame until it glows red. After the needle has cooled, gently puncture the blister at its outer edge, and press to force fluid out. Do not remove the skin covering the blister. Protect with a small bandage.

• **Redness and swelling around a blister** indicate infection, particularly if there are red streaks and a discharge of yellowish pus. Consult a physician.

BURSITIS: *See SHOULDER PAIN*

Charley Horse: *See MUSCLE SPASM OR CRAMP*

CHEST PAIN. Pain in parts of the chest may have a variety of causes. Some, such as indigestion, are relatively harmless. Others may be caused or aggravated by exercise: muscle soreness, inflammation of the rib cartilage, rib fracture or poor breathing. Still others may be an indication of heart trouble.

• **A steady ache or stabbing pain on one side of the chest** can be caused by TEARS or SPASMS of the chest muscles or the muscles between the shoulder blades. Massage, heat or correcting posture by regularly stretching the muscles around your spine *(page 95)* generally bring relief.

If you feel pain in the middle of the chest, you may have developed a SWOLLEN CARTILAGE between your ribs and your breastbone. No special treatment is needed; the condition will subside with rest and time.

• **A constant dull pain that becomes very sharp** when you breathe is an indication of a CRACKED RIB caused by a sudden fall, blow or twist. You can treat it by wearing a constricting canvas band around your ribs for three to four weeks.

• **Viselike constricting pain,** centered over the front of the chest but sometimes felt in the abdomen or shoulders, is the most common indication of HEART TROUBLE, and always calls for medical attention. The pain may radiate down the left arm, across the chest, to the shoulder or into the neck. It may be accompanied by weakness or sweating. Two additional indications will help you to identify heart pain: It is generally eased by sitting up, not by lying down; and it is rarely so localized that you can cover the pain with one finger. If such a pain subsides after about 10 minutes of rest, consult a physician, but you can wait until the next day. If it does not subside quickly, get medical attention immediately.

CRAMPS: *See MUSCLE SPASM OR CRAMP*

Elbow Pain. A pain in the region of the elbow, particularly where the forearm muscles are attached to the bone just below the elbow joint, is a sign of TENDINITIS, inflammation of the tendons— the fibrous bands of tissue that connect a muscle to a bone. The ailment is commonly called tennis elbow *(page 136),* but people

who have never held a racket can suffer from it. Any motion that stresses the tendons in the area of the elbow, such as throwing a ball, bowling or putting the shot, can strain and inflame these tendons.

• **Elbow pain following exercise** generally disappears with rest. Do not play tennis or otherwise stress the forearm until the pain is completely gone. When your forearm is free of pain, you can strengthen its muscles by lifting weights or by swinging the racket with the cover on. You can avoid tennis elbow by adjusting the motions you use in the exercise that caused it—in tennis, for example, a backhand stroke made with a rigid wrist and a locked elbow generally prevents tendon injury.

If elbow pain persists, with swelling or reddening, a tendon may be torn. Consult a physician at your convenience.

Foot Pain. Pain in a foot may be confined to a single area or felt throughout the entire foot. It may arise in extended walking or running exercise, or in sports that require you to make sudden twists and changes of position.

• **Pain in the arches** is generally caused by muscle strain. It will usually be relieved if you stop running for two or three days and change to cushioned, well-fitting shoes.

• **Exercise-induced pain at the base of a big toe** is generally the result of a bruise and should respond to rest alone.

• **Pain in the sole or heel** at the site of the thickened, hardened patch of a callus is a certain sign of ill-fitting shoes. The cure is a properly fitted pair with cushioned soles and heels.

• **General pain throughout the foot** may be more serious. Press gently on the foot from both above and below simultaneously; if you feel additional pain with this kind of pressure, you may have a STRESS FRACTURE, a hairline crack in the surface of a foot bone. Such a fracture will generally heal by itself if you rest the foot.

If general pain persists for more than a week, consult a physician; you may have a large stress fracture—an injury that needs professional treatment.

FROSTBITE: *See SKIN NUMB AND WHITE*

Groin Ringworm: *See ITCHY GROIN*

Heart Irregularity. During exercise the heart beats faster than its normal rate of 72 to 78 beats per minute. The increase is normal, and generally indicates a healthy heart.

• **A heart rate exceeding 100 beats per minute and also fluttering** generally indicates temporary TACHYCARDIA, common among people beginning to exercise strenuously. The heart rate slows and the beat steadies when you end the exercise session, and the fluttering disappears entirely as fitness improves.

● **An uncomfortably rapid and wildly fluctuating heartbeat** that comes on in a sudden rush during exercise and subsides only after considerable rest may be a sign of ARRHYTHMIA. It may be harmless but it may also indicate heart trouble; if you experience arrhythmia even after reaching a high level of fitness, consult a physician.

● **A slower-than-normal resting pulse rate** is common among those in especially good physical condition. In such people, a heart rate below 60 beats per minute at rest is a good sign and no cause for alarm; it indicates a heart muscle with plenty of reserve strength.

HEART TROUBLE: *See CHEST PAIN*
HEAT EXHAUSTION: *See SKIN CHILLED AND DAMP*
HEAT PROSTRATION: *See SKIN CHILLED AND DAMP*
HEATSTROKE: *See SKIN DRY AND HOT*

HEEL PAIN. Pain under the heel bone may be due to a simple bruise caused by exercising in thin-soled shoes on hard surfaces or on surfaces containing sharp rocks and pebbles. A bruise should need only several days of rest to heal.

If pain under the heel spreads along the bottom of the foot or is accompanied by a bump either on the bottom of the heel or at the point where the heel meets the Achilles tendon, you may have PLANTAR FASCIITIS, a tear and inflammation of the tissues called fasciae, which protect nerves and muscles. Rest, soaking in warm water and massage are the best treatments; if the pain persists, consult a foot doctor. This ailment is caused by pressure, pounding or a sudden unexpected turn, and it can generally be prevented by well-cushioned and flexible shoes *(pages 76-77)*.

HEEL SPUR OR BUMP: *See HEEL PAIN*
HEEL TENDON PAIN: *See ACHILLES TENDON PAIN*

HIP PAIN. Few types of pain are as varied in degree or origin as those of the hip. Pain can be localized or can radiate from either or both of the hips into the lower back or down the leg, and it may originate from problems located outside the hip—in the lower back or in the knee, leg or foot.

● **Hip pain that radiates from the hip** to the back of the thigh and leg, often called SCIATICA, may be due to an unstable lower spine or to a ruptured spinal disc. Pain from these causes may be relieved by rest; if it persists, consult a physician.

● **Hip pain that is felt upon any motion,** usually with tenderness over part of the hip, is generally caused by inflammation. Apply an ice pack to the hip at least twice a day for 30-minute periods,

allowing 15-minute intervals between applications. You may apply the ice pack as often as you wish. If pain and swelling persist after one or two days of treatment, consult a physician.

● **Hip pain that is felt only when the hip is bearing weight,** especially in running, is generally caused by a STRESS FRACTURE. Do not run until pain in the foot and hip is relieved. If pain is still severe after a week, consult a physician.

● **Hip pain in the hip opposite to the one bearing weight** may result from a minor difference in the lengths of the legs, or it may be caused by a knee injury.

If you have hurt your knee and pain and swelling have not gone down after several hours, consult a physician. The hip pain can be relieved only by correcting the knee problem.

If you have not hurt your knee, compare leg lengths by standing erect in your bare feet while someone places his hands, palms down, around the crests of your pelvic bone; the hand on the shorter side will be seen to be lower. If you see such a difference, consult a physician for an accurate measurement and, if necessary, a prescription for a shoe heel lift to compensate.

● **Hip pain that is present only during exercise** is generally caused by FLAT or OVERPRONATED FEET *(page 137)*, which roll the ankle inward. Shoes with arch supports may relieve the pain; if they do not, consult a foot doctor, who can prescribe a removable shoe support called an orthotic to correct the balance of your feet.

HYPOTHERMIA: *See SPEECH SLURRING*

INDIGESTION: *See STITCH IN THE SIDE*
INFECTION: *See SKIN IRRITATION and SKIN SCRAPES*

ITCHING FEET. Itchiness, scaling and dryness, usually beginning in the spaces between the third and fourth toes and sometimes spreading to the soles, signal athlete's foot, an infection by a fungus called ringworm. In hot weather the ailment may flare up into red, cracking, painful sores; infected toenails may become thickened and distorted in shape. Apply fungicide containing micronazole nitrate or undecylenic acid, available at drugstores. If you are susceptible to this fungal infection, take steps to keep it from attacking you in the first place. Do not walk barefoot in a swimming-pool area or locker room, where the disease is easily transmitted. Keep your feet as dry as possible by exposing them to air and by powdering them regularly with talcum powder. Always dry your feet thoroughly after bathing, and change socks frequently.

If athlete's foot resists home treatment, consult a physician. The fungus infection sometimes proves difficult to eradicate, and it may be complicated by bacterial infection.

ITCHY GROIN. A red, sometimes flaky rash, often accompanied by ring-shaped markings in the groin area and the inner parts of the upper thighs, is common among male exercisers. Colloquially called jock itch, it is caused by a fungus that generally can be eliminated by nonprescription medications containing micronazole nitrate or tolnaflate (look on the label), provided treatment is continued faithfully for the time recommended.

Do not wear tight clothing, which can irritate and worsen the condition. If the infection persists, consult a dermatologist.

JOCK ITCH: *See ITCHY GROIN*

KNEECAP PAIN. Pain behind the kneecap during exercise, often called runner's knee *(page 137),* is most frequently caused by FLAT FEET or by OVERPRONATION—rolling of the foot too far inward at each stride. In both conditions, treat the pain by temporarily stopping the exercise. To avoid recurrence, wear well-made, properly fitted running shoes *(pages 76-77),* to which arch supports, available at shoe stores, have been added.

LUMBAGO: *See BACK PAIN*

MAT BURN: *See SKIN SCRAPES*

MENSTRUAL IRREGULARITY. Women who exercise vigorously for considerable lengths of time, particularly in training for competition, may skip their monthly periods. Such AMENORRHEA is usually caused by the emotional stress of intense training, but it can also result from crash dieting, overweight, glandular disorders, and serious illnesses such as diabetes and tuberculosis.

If your monthly periods cease, ease up on your training schedules and dieting. Because fertility may continue in the absence of menstruation, do not make any change in birth-control measures. If a slowdown in training regime or a return to more normal eating patterns has no effect, consult a physician.

MORTON'S FOOT: *See TOE PAIN*

MUSCLE SPASM OR CRAMP. Most such pains are simply the results of unaccustomed exercise and fatigue, and disappear with rest and gentle massage of the afflicted area. The sore muscles are usually swollen and tender, and in the legs may contain microscopic tears called SHIN SPLINTS.

• **Cramps marked by painful involuntary contractions of the muscles** may arise from exercising in high heat and humidity, which leads to fatigue, sudden temperature change and a deficiency of salt. Gentle massage may aggravate such cramps, but a drink of very lightly salted water and a rest may relieve them.

• **A very severe cramp** may be caused by a sudden strain or tearing of an entire muscle. Treat it by resting the afflicted limb, by a local application of ice and by compression and elevation *(see ANKLE PAIN).* If the tear is small, with slight pain, gentle active stretching after 12 to 24 hours also helps. If pain persists, consult a physician. Avoid active exercise until you are free from pain through the normal range of motion.

• **A spasm,** especially in the muscles of the front of the thigh, sometimes called a Charley horse, is a severe cramp that can come from a fall or overstretching a muscle or tendon. Push your foot against resistance, such as the hand of a helper, until the leg is fully extended. Avoid deep massage, which may cause calcium compounds to stiffen the muscle tissue.

NAUSEA: *See SKIN CHILLED AND DAMP and SKIN DRY AND HOT*

RINGWORM: *See ITCHY GROIN*
RUNNER'S KNEE: *See KNEECAP PAIN*

SCIATICA: *See HIP PAIN*

SHIN PAIN. Pain along the shins and calves, common among runners and those who run as part of a sport, is usually caused by microscopic muscle tears called SHIN SPLINTS. The immediate cause is generally overtilting, or overpronating, the feet while running *(page 137).* Rest, ice packs, compression and elevation *(see ANKLE PAIN)* will ease the pain. Do not run again until the pain has largely disappeared, and before resuming running, strengthen the muscles of the calves with exercises of the kind shown on pages 102 and 107. During the healing period, which may last up to two months, run only on grass. Arch supports, available at drugstores, may help prevent recurrence.

If mild shin pain persists throughout the healing period, consult a physician.

If shin pain is more than a nuisance and persists for more than two weeks, consult a physician. Such pain may be caused by a crack in the shin bone rather than by injured muscles.

SHIN SPLINTS: *See MUSCLE SPASM OR CRAMP and SHIN PAIN*

SHOULDER PAIN. Pain in one or both shoulders, common among those who use their arms vigorously while exercising or participating in sports, is generally caused by BURSITIS, an inflammation of fluid-filled sacs, called bursae, that cushion the moving parts of a joint.

If shoulder pain follows exercise, rest the shoulder by stopping all activities that require the action used to hit or throw a ball, but maintain a light routine of strengthening exercises.

● **Shoulder pain accompanied by swelling, tenderness and muscle weakness** may be due to CHRONIC BURSITIS, in which the walls of one or more bursae are thickened and the lining has degenerated. Consult a physician, but you can wait until the next day.

SKIN CHILLED AND DAMP. Cold, pale skin and profuse sweating, which may be accompanied by weakness, dizziness, nausea and dim or blurred vision, can be a sign of HEAT PROSTRATION. It generally results from the body's temporary inability to adjust to one of its own natural responses to heat—the expansion of the blood vessels just under the skin—and does not usually require medical care. Stop exercising and lie or sit down in a cool place; loosen your clothing. Drink cool (not icy cold) water. If you do not feel better after an hour or so, or if you have dry, hot skin and blurred vision that do not improve with rest, you may have HEATSTROKE. See *SKIN DRY AND HOT.*

SKIN DRY AND HOT. Dry, hot skin, accompanied by a sudden rise in body temperature to 105° F. or more, is a warning sign of impending HEATSTROKE, which can be fatal and always requires immediate medical attention. To avoid heatstroke, do not exercise during the extremes of temperature and humidity indicated in the chart on page 74.

If the only symptoms are dry, hot skin and fever, stop exercising immediately and lie down, either in the shade outdoors or in a cool, ventilated place indoors.

If the basic symptoms are accompanied by labored breathing, a dry mouth and a muscular twitching or cramps, blurred vision, nausea, disjointed thinking, convulsions or unconsciousness, the victim should be given first aid immediately and medical attention as quickly as possible thereafter. Soak the victim's body in a cold bath, or cover it with a blanket soaked in cold water and massage the victim's chilled skin until the body temperature falls. Do not continue to chill the victim after reducing the body temperature to less than 102° F., but be sure you get professional help.

SKIN IRRITATION. Red, tender skin over a broad, slightly swollen area may be caused by simple chafing, an allergy or infection. The main differences in symptoms are in the degree of swelling.

● **Mild redness and tenderness,** with little or no swelling, indicates chafed skin. The most common causes are tight clothing, especially at the groin or under the arms, and the rubbing of a seam, a coarse stitch or a fastener; sensitive areas such as the nipples are more likely to be irritated, and perspiration aggravates the tendency of all skin to chafe. Application of petroleum jelly or baby powder helps. To prevent further irritation, choose clothes that are roomy, loosely woven and well ventilated. Synthetic fabrics are less apt to irritate the skin than cotton or wool because they create less friction and dry more quickly when soaked with perspiration, but they tend to retard the evaporation of perspiration.

● **Redness accompanied by general swelling,** and sometimes by itching, may be caused by dyes that stimulate an allergic reaction in the skin; the offending clothing or equipment can usually be identified from the pattern or location of the red swelling. With repeated exposure the skin may "weep" and the surface break down. If you suspect that you have an allergy, consult a physician.

● **A localized red, tender swelling** of the skin may indicate an infection, which can start from the irritation of a hair follicle by sweat and by clothing that chafes the skin. If you suspect an infection, consult a physician.

SKIN NUMB AND WHITE. Exercising outdoors in very cold weather, particularly if there is air movement from wind or from the speed of your cycling or skiing, may lead to frostbite. Blood vessels freeze solid, and blood does not circulate; the lack of circulating blood whitens the frostbitten area. Because frostbite can cause permanent harm, do not exercise outdoors if the combination of temperature and wind reaches dangerous levels *(page 74)*.

● **A pain in the face, ears, fingers or toes in cold weather,** especially if spots of white appear, indicates frostbite. Do not attempt to thaw a frostbite outdoors; a refrozen area is more dangerous than the original frostbite. Go indoors immediately. For mild frostbite, simply stay indoors in a warm room until the frozen skin thaws. As the frostbitten area regains circulation, the skin will become bright red and painful. If a frostbite does not respond to this treatment, consult a physician immediately.

SKIN SCRAPES. Called a "mat burn" by wrestlers, a "strawberry" by baseball players, a skin abrasion is generally harmless but should be protected against infection.

If the skin is simply reddened and scratched, wash it gently with soap and water, dry with a clean towel and cover with a gauze pad and adhesive tape.

If an abrasion swells, treat as above but also apply an antibiotic ointment containing polymixin or bacitracin; such ointments are available without prescription at drugstores.

If an untreated abrasion has developed yellowish-white pus on or just beneath the surface of the skin, you have contracted an infection. Consult a physician.

SLIPPED OR RUPTURED DISC: *See BACK PAIN*

SPEECH SLURRING. During outdoor exercise in cold weather, the inability to enunciate clearly, numb fingers and shivering are signs of HYPOTHERMIA. This is a potentially fatal condition, marked by a drop in body temperature and, in its late stages, requiring immediate medical attention; if the body temperature drops 23 degrees or more below normal, the heart will stop pumping. Go indoors immediately and take a warm (not hot) bath. If a victim of hypothermia lapses into unconsciousness, get him to a hospital emergency room as quickly as possible.

STITCH IN THE SIDE. A sudden, sharp pain in the upper abdomen, common in exercising, particularly among runners, is a form of muscle cramp generally due to indigestion or, according to some theories, to poor circulation in the chest muscles. Gas in the intestinal tract, the most likely cause, distends, and triggers spasms in, the colon. To relieve a stitch, stop exercising and rest, breathing as deeply as you can until the pain disappears. To avoid future cramps, do not exercise soon after eating — a wait of three to five hours may be advisable if you are to engage in prolonged, strenuous exertion. Also maintain bowel regularity, using laxatives if necessary. If cramps persist, consult a physician at your convenience.

STRAWBERRY: *See SKIN SCRAPES*
STRESS FRACTURE: *See FOOT PAIN and HIP PAIN*
SWELLING: *See SKIN IRRITATION and SKIN SCRAPES*

TACHYCARDIA: *See HEART IRREGULARITY*
TENNIS ELBOW: *See ELBOW PAIN*

TOE PAIN. If you regularly suffer shooting pain between or in your toes, particularly the third and fourth toes, examine your feet to see whether the big toe is shorter than the second. A short big toe can unbalance the foot, causing overpronation *(page 137)* or causing the other toes to hurt during exercise. Massage may relieve the pain; arch supports and heel lifts, which are available in pharmacies and athletic supply stores, may help prevent it. For stubborn cases, consult a foot doctor.

UNCONSCIOUSNESS OR COMA: *See SKIN DRY AND HOT and SPEECH SLURRING*

Bibliography

BOOKS

Ahuja, Savitri, *Savitri's Way to Perfect Fitness through Hatha Yoga*. Simon and Schuster, 1979.

American Medical Association, *Standard Nomenclature of Athletic Injuries*. 1976.

Anderson, Bob, *Stretching*. Shelter Publications, 1980.

Åstrand, Per-Olof, and Kaare Rodahl, *Textbook of Work Physiology*. McGraw-Hill, 1977.

Brems, Marianne, *Swim for Fitness*. Chronicle, 1979.

Calhoun, Michael F., *The Parcourse Guide to Fitness*. Parcourse, Ltd., 1979.

Clarke, H. Harrison, *Application of Measurement to Health and Physical Education*. Prentice-Hall, 1976.

Clarke, H. Harrison, and David H. Clarke, *Developmental and Adapted Physical Education*. Prentice-Hall, 1978.

Cooper, Kenneth H.: *Aerobics*. Bantam, 1968. *The New Aerobics*. Bantam, 1976.

Costill, David L., *A Scientific Approach to Distance Running*. Track & Field News, 1979.

Cureton, Thomas K., Jr., *Physical Fitness and Dynamic Health*. Dial Press, 1973.

DeVries, Herbert A.: *Physiology of Exercise*. Wm. C. Brown, 1980. *Vigor Regained*. Prentice-Hall, 1980.

Dominguez, Richard H., *The Complete Book of Sports Medicine*. Scribner's Sons, 1979.

Edington, D. W., and V. R. Edgerton, *The Biology of Physical Activity*. Houghton Mifflin, 1976.

Fox, Edward L., *Sports Physiology*. Saunders, 1979.

Glover, Bob, and Jack Shepherd, *The Runner's Handbook*. Penguin, 1978.

Jacobson, Howard, *Racewalk to Fitness*. Simon and Schuster, 1980.

Katch, Frank I., and William D. McArdle, *Nutrition, Weight Control, and Exercise*. Houghton Mifflin, 1977.

Katch, Frank I., et al., *Getting in Shape*. Houghton Mifflin, 1979.

Kraus, Hans, *Backache Stress and Tension*. Simon and Schuster, 1965.

Kuntzleman, Charles T., *Rating the Exercises*. William Morrow, 1978.

Lamb, David R., *Physiology of Exercise*. Macmillan, 1978.

Lehninger, Albert L., *Biochemistry*. Worth Publishers, 1976.

Man-ch'ing, Cheng, and Robert W. Smith, *T'ai-Chi: The "Supreme Ultimate" Exercise for Health, Sport, and Self-Defense*.

Charles E. Tuttle, 1974.

Mathews, Donald K., and Edward L. Fox, *The Physiological Basis of Physical Education and Athletics*. Saunders, 1976.

Mirkin, Gabe, and Marshall Hoffman, *The Sportsmedicine Book*. Little, Brown, 1978.

Myers, Clayton R., *The Official YMCA Physical Fitness Handbook*. Popular Library, 1975.

Percival, Jan, et al., *The Complete Guide to Total Fitness*. Methuen, 1977.

The Rand McNally Atlas of the Body and Mind. Rand McNally, 1976.

Rasch, Philip J., and Roger K. Burke, *Kinesiology and Applied Anatomy*. Lea & Febiger, 1978.

Rosen, Gerald, *The Relaxation Book*. Prentice-Hall, 1977.

Sheehan, George A.: *Dr. George Sheehan's Medical Advice for Runners*. World Publications, 1978. *Dr. Sheehan on Running*. Bantam, 1978.

Stryer, Lubert, *Biochemistry*. W. H. Freeman, 1975.

Vander, Arthur J., et al., *Human Physiology: The Mechanisms of Body Function*. McGraw-Hill, 1980.

White, John, and James Fadiman, eds., *Relax: How You Can Feel Better, Reduce Stress and Overcome Tension*. Confucian Press, 1976.

Zohman, Lenore R., et al., *The Cardiologists' Guide to Fitness and Health through Exercise*. Simon and Schuster, 1979.

PERIODICALS

Adams, William C., et al., "Effects of Equivalent Sea-Level and Altitude Training on VO₂max and Running Performance." *Journal of Applied Physiology*, August 1975.

Brown, Robert S., et al., "The Prescription of Exercise for Depression." *The Physician and Sportsmedicine*, December 1978.

Costill, David L., "Muscle Exhaustion." *The Physician and Sportsmedicine*, October 1974.

Costill, D. L., and B. Saltin, "Factors Limiting Gastric Emptying during Rest and Exercise." *Journal of Applied Physiology*, November 1974.

DeVries, Herbert A., and Gene M. Adams, "Electromyographic Comparison of Single Doses of Exercise and Meprobamate as to Effects on Muscular Relaxation." *American Journal of Physical Medicine*, June 1972.

Dimsdale, Joel E., and Jonathan Moss, "Plasma Catecholamines in Stress and Exercise." *Journal of the American Medical Association*, January 25, 1980.

Ellestad, M. H., et al., "Stress Testing: Clinical Application and Predictive Capacity." *Progress in Cardiovascular Diseases*, May-June 1979.

"Exercise and the Cardiovascular System." *The Physician and Sportsmedicine*, September 1979.

"Exercise, Not Diet, Determines HDL Levels." *The Physician and Sportsmedicine*, December 1978.

Fortuin, Nicholas J., and James L. Weiss, "Exercise Stress Testing." *Circulation*, November 1977.

Gollnick, Philip D., et al., "The Muscle Biopsy: Still a Research Tool." *The Physician and Sportsmedicine*, January 1980.

Greist, John H., et al., "Running out of Depression." *The Physician and Sportsmedicine*, December 1978.

Kalenak, Alexander, et al., "Athletic Injuries: Heat vs. Cold." *American Family Physician*, November 1975.

Martin, Jack: "Corporate Health: A Result of Employee Fitness." *The Physician and Sportsmedicine*, March 1978. "In Activity Therapy, Patients Literally Move toward Mental Health." *The Physician and Sportsmedicine*, July 1977.

Marx, Jean L., "The HDL: The Good Cholesterol Carriers?" *Science*, August 1979.

"Old Runners Overtake the Aging Process." *Medical World News*, April 30, 1979.

Paffenbarger, R. S., Jr., et al., "Current Exercise and Heart Attack Risk." *Cardiac Rehabilitation*, summer 1979.

Pattengale, Paul K., and John O. Holloszy, "Augmentation of Skeletal Muscle Myoglobin in a Program of Treadmill Running." *Journal of Physiology*, September 1967.

Pipes, Thomas V., and Jack H. Wilmore, "Isokinetic vs Isotonic Strength Training in Adult Men." *Medicine and Science in Sports*, winter 1975.

Rode, Andris, and Roy J. Shephard, "The Influence of Cigarette Smoking upon the Oxygen Cost of Breathing in Near-Maximal Exercise." *Medicine and Science in Sports*, summer 1971.

Rynearson, Robert R., et al., "Do Physician Athletes Believe in Pre-Exercise Examinations and Stress Tests?" *The New England Journal of Medicine*, October 4, 1979.

Siegel, Arthur J., et al., "Paternal History of Coronary-Heart Disease Reported by Marathon Runners." *The New England*

Journal of Medicine, July 12, 1979.
''Strenuous Sports Better for Heart, MD Reports.'' *The Physician and Sportsmedicine,* January 1978.
Weiner, J. S., and M. Khogali, ''A Physiological Body-Cooling Unit for Treatment of Heat Stroke.'' *The Lancet,* March 8, 1980.
Wilmore, Jack H., ''Alterations in Strength, Body Composition and Anthropometric Measurements Consequent to a 10-Week Weight Training Program.'' *Medicine and Science in Sports,* summer 1974.

OTHER PUBLICATIONS
The Perrier Study: Fitness in America. Louis Harris and Associates, Inc., January 1979.

Picture credits

The sources for the illustrations that appear in this book are listed below. Credits for the illustrations from left to right are separated by semicolons, from top to bottom by dashes.

Cover: Henry Groskinsky. 7: Albrecht Gaebele, Pfedelbach. 8: © Field Enterprises Inc., 1950, courtesy of Harry S. Truman Library. 10: Memorial Hall at South Dakota State Historical Society. 13: Copied by Steve Altman. 14, 15: Courtesy Food and Drug Administration; copied by Steve Altman; courtesy Robert A. Skufca from the Food and Drug Administration. 16: From *The Unfashionable Human Body* by Bernard Rudofsky, published by Doubleday & Company, Inc., 1971, inset, Library of Congress. 17: © Bob Adelman. 19: Al Freni, courtesy Fairfax County Fire and Rescue Services. 21: Harold Elrick, M.D., Director of Foundation for Optimal Health and Longevity— David Hiser. 23: Dieter Heggemann from *Stern,* Hamburg. 24, 25: Baldev from Sygma. 26: Fred Ward from Black Star. 27: Rene Burri from Magnum. 28, 29: © LISL '75, Image Bank; Elliot Erwitt from Magnum. 30: Alain Nogues from Sygma. 31: © Paolo Koch from Photo Researchers. 32, 33: Al Freni. 35: *The Champ,* reprinted by permission of Estate of Norman Rockwell and *The Saturday Evening Post,* © 1922, The Curtis Publishing Co. 36: T/Sgt. Ruth M. Heeler, U.S. Air Force. 37: Courtesy of Per-Olof Åstrand, Stockholm. 39: Fil Hunter. 41: Charles Atlas, Ltd., of New York. 42: Bruce W. Most. 44-47: Walter E.

Hilmers Jr., HJ Commercial Art. 49: Fil Hunter. 50: J. Aronson, 1978, *The Daily Telegraph* from Woodfin Camp and Associates, inset, Jerry Cooke from *Sports Illustrated.* 52, 53: Bundesarchiv, Koblenz. 54: Smith College Archives; Bettmann Archives, Inc. 55: Byron Collection, Museum of the City of New York. 56, 57: National Council of Young Men's Christian Associations. 58, 59: I.N.R.P. Musée de l'Education, Rouen; Culver Pictures, Inc. 60: Ullstein Bilderdienst, Berlin (West). 61: NCR Corporation. 62, 63: Library of Congress. 65: Enrico Ferorelli. 67-69: © John Blaustein, 1979. 71: © 1979 David Madison from *Runner's World Magazine.* 72-77: Walter E. Hilmers Jr., HJ Commercial Art. 80, 81: Photo by Henry Groskinsky, drawings by Frederic F. Bigio from B-C Graphics. 83: Courtesy Professor Dr. Josef Keul, Medizinische Universitätsklinik, Freiburg. 85-88: Enrico Ferorelli. 92-112: Fil Hunter. 113: Walter E. Hilmers Jr., HJ Commercial Art. 115: Jane Sobel from © Janeart, 1980. 117: Charlie Doyle from Runner's Image. 118: Lane Stewart from *Sports Illustrated.* 120: Gerald R. Brimacombe from *Sports Illustrated.* 121: Andrew S. Novick from Photo-on-Wheels. 123: © Marvin Newman from Woodfin Camp and Associates. 124: Ted Spiegel from Black Star; © Paolo Koch from Photo Researchers. 125: John Launois from Black Star — Joop Fenstra, Leeuwarden, Holland. 126: Walter E. Hilmers Jr., HJ Commercial Art. 129: Art Seitz. 130: Photo Benoist Collignon from Agence S.A.M., Paris — Stanley Paul, Ltd., from *Football Fitness* by Bill Watson, courtesy *Strength and Health.* 131: Colorsport, London. 132: *Dallas Cowboys Weekly.* 134: UPI; Smith College Archives. 136, 137: Jane Gordon. 139: Lanny Johnson, inset, Dyonics, Inc. 141, 143: Library of Congress. 145: © Lennart Nilsson from *Behold Man,* Little, Brown and Co., 1974. 147: Dr. Ray Clark and M. R. Goff from Science Photo Library, London. 148: P. D. Gollnick. 151: Photo by Dr. Harold Edgerton, MIT, art from *Biochemistry* by Lubert Stryer, W. H. Freeman and Company, © 1975. 152, 154: Photos by Edweard J. Muybridge for International Museum of Photography at George Eastman House, details from Animal Locomotion, plates No. 60 and No. 323. 156: Russel Munson. 157: P. D. Gollnick. 158: Joan S. McGurren. 159: Caruso of Montreal. 160, 161: Rex E. Carrow from College of Human Medicine, Michigan State University, diagrams by Joan S. McGurren. 162, 163: Armed Forces Institute of Pathology, diagram by Joan S.

McGurren. 164, 165: Armed Forces Institute of Pathology, except top left, diagram by Joan S. McGurren.

Acknowledgments

The index for this book was prepared by Barbara L. Klein. For their valuable help with the preparation of this volume, the editors wish to thank the following: Dr. David M. Brody, Washington, D.C.; Dr. Rex Carrow, Michigan State University, East Lansing, Mich.; David L. Costill, Ball State University, Muncie, Ind.; Dr. James E. Counsilman, Indiana University, Bloomington, Ind.; Emily A. Craig, Hughston Sports Medicine Foundation, Inc., Columbus, Ga.; Dr. Nathan Dean, Salt Lake Emergency Physicians, Salt Lake City, Utah; Dr. Samuel M. Fox III, Georgetown University Medical Center, Washington, D.C.; Ramiro A. Galindo, Bryan, Tex.; Elise M. Giebel, Bethesda, Md.; Dr. Lawrence A. Golding, University of Nevada at Las Vegas; Dr. Philip D. Gollnick, Washington State University at Pullman; Dr. Joe Griffin, Armed Forces Institute of Pathology, Washington, D.C.; Steve Hornor, Washington Diplomats Soccer Club, Washington, D.C.; Ken Jones, Fairfax County Fire and Rescue Services, Fairfax, Va.; Dr. Richard Jones, Georgetown University Medical Center, Washington, D.C.; Shinzo Kobori, Brookings Institution, Washington, D.C.; Lawrence B. Krause, Brookings Institution, Washington, D.C.; Clifford Kress, Dyonics, Inc., Woburn, Mass.; Dr. Fritz Lipmann, The Rockefeller University in New York; Dr. H. Carroll Parish, Santa Monica, Calif.; Gayle Pierson, Alexandria YMCA in Va.; President's Council on Physical Fitness and Sports, Washington, D.C.; Edwin O. Reischauer, Harvard University, Cambridge, Mass.; Charles Rule, Fairfax County Fire and Rescue Services, Fairfax, Va.; *Runner's World Magazine,* Mountain View, Calif.; *Running Times,* Woodbridge, Va.; Dr. Myles J. Schneider, Annandale, Va.; James H. Sherman, University of Michigan Medical School at Ann Arbor; Dr. Robert Skufca, Food and Drug Administration, Silver Spring, Md.; Dr. Steven I. Subotnick, Hayward, Calif.; Mary Trott, Smith College Archives, Northampton, Mass.; Coralee Van Egmond, National Jogging Association, Washington, D.C.; Thomas A. Ziebarth, U.S. Postal Service's Consumer Protection Office, Washington, D.C.

Index